Math *for* Nurses

A Pocket Guide to
Dosage Calculation and
Drug Preparation

FIFTH EDITION

FIFTH EDITION

Math *for* Nurses

A Pocket Guide to
Dosage Calculation and
Drug Preparation

Mary Jo Boyer, R.N., D.N.Sc.
Coadjutant Nursing Faculty
Former Dean and Professor of Nursing and Allied Health
Delaware County Community College
Media, Pennsylvania

Consultant
Elaine Dreisbaugh, B.S.N., M.S.N., C.P.N.P
Assistant Professor of Nursing
Delaware County Community College
Media, Pennsylvania
Nurse Educator, The Chester County Hospital
West Chester, Pennsylvania

 Lippincott
Philadelphia · New York · Baltimore

Acquisitions Editor: Margaret Zuccarini
Sponsoring Editor: Helen Kogut
Senior Project Editor: Sandra Cherrey Scheinin
Senior Production Manager: Helen Ewan
Production Coordinator: Nannette Winski
Design Coordinator: Brett MacNaughton
Interior Designer: Holly Reid McLaughlin
Cover Designer: Melissa Walter
Manufacturing Manager: William Alberti
Compositor: Peirce Graphic Services
Printer: R.R. Donnelley & Sons, Crawfordsville

Edition 5th

Library of Congress Cataloging-in Publication Data
Boyer, Mary Jo.
    Math for nurses : a pocket guide in dosage calculation and drug preparation / Mary Jo Boyer.—5th ed.
        p. cm.
    Includes index.
    ISBN 0-7817-3468-1 (alk. paper)
    1. Nursing—Mathematics—Handbooks, manuals, etc.
2. Pharmaceutical arithmetic—Handbooks, manuals, etc. I. Title.

RT68 .B68 2002
615′.14—dc21

                                          2001029925

To

The nursing and allied health faculty and students at Delaware County Community College who have inspired and supported my writing since 1982.

To

Carol Lillis, Dean of Nursing and Allied Health, whose friendship over 25 years, has enriched my professional and personal life.

Reviewers

Susan Buchholz, RN, BSN, MSN
Assistant Professor, Nursing Department
Georgia Perimeter College
Clarkston, Georgia

Cornelia Gordon, BSN, BA, MA
Nursing Instructor
McLennan Community College
Waco, Texas

Victoria Lynne Oxner, RN, MSN
Practical Nursing Chair/Instructor
Arkansas State University Mountain Home
Mountain Home, Arkansas

Joan B. Winkle, RN, MSN
Faculty of Nursing
Alabama Southern Community College
Monroeville, Alabama

Preface

The idea for this compact, pocket-sized book about dosage calculation was generated by my students. For several years I watched as they took their math-related handouts and photocopied them, reducing them to a size that would fit into the pockets of their uniforms or laboratory coats. This "pocket" reference material was readily accessible when a math calculation was needed to administer a drug. Each year the number of papers that were copied increased as each group of students passed on their ideas to the next group. I also noted that staff nurses were using this readily available and compact information as a reference for math problems.

When a student then asked: "Why not put together for us all the information that we need?" I thought, "Why not?" The idea was born, the commitment made, and 18 months later the first edition of *Math for Nurses* was published in 1987. It is my hope that it will continue, in this fifth edition, to be helpful to all who need a quick reference source when struggling with dosage calculations and drug preparation.

ORGANIZATION

This pocket guide is divided into three units to facilitate quick access to specific information needed to administer drugs. The preassessment test should be completed before reading Chapter 1 to determine the basic level of math ability. Unit I presents a review of basic math, starting with the fundamentals of Roman and Arabic numerals. Chapters 3 and 4 cover common and decimal fractions. Chapter 5 shows you how to set up a ratio and proportion and solve for *x,* using a colon or fraction format. It also uses drug-related word problems as examples to help you solve for *x.* This information is essential, a foundation for understanding the dosage calculations presented in Unit III.

Unit II focuses on the metric system, the apothecaries' system, and household units of measurement. Chapter 9 lists system equivalents and shows you how to convert from one unit of measurement to another. Some of these system equivalents are duplicated on the inside front cover to provide easy and quick access when calculating drug problems.

Unit III, the most comprehensive and detailed section of this pocket guide, contains Medication Labels, a new chapter with this edition. The chapter explains how to read and interpret medication labels, with sample questions provided for reinforcement. Chapters 11 and 12 cover oral and parenteral dosage problems where pediatric doses have been incorporated. Throughout this unit, problem-solving methodology is presented in a simple, easy-to-follow manner. A step-by-step approach is used, which will guide the reader through each set of examples.

✚ NEW CONTENT

For this edition, each unit now concludes with End of Unit Review questions. An additional 140 new questions have been added, per students' requests, to provide more practice in problem solving. A new appendix, Dimensional Analysis, has been added and includes a step-by-step process to use for solving drug dosage calculations. Two sample problems have been included in this appendix. A laminated card, containing volume and weight equivalents and dosage calculations formulas, has been added for easy quick reference.

Math for Nurses was written for all nurses who administer drugs. It is intended as a quick, easy, and readily accessible guide when dosage calculations are required. It is my hope that its use will help nurses to calculate dosages accurately and, as a result, to improve the accuracy of drug delivery.

It is our inherent responsibility as nurses to ensure that every patient entrusted to our care receives the correct dosage of medication delivered in the most appropriate way.

Mary Jo Boyer, R.N., D.N.SC.

How to Use This Book

This book is designed for two purposes:

- To help you learn how to calculate drug dosages and administer medications.
- To serve as a quick reference when reinforcement of learning is required.

The best way to use this pocket guide is to:

- Read the rules and examples.
- Follow the steps for solving the problems.
- Work the practice problems.
- Write down your answers and notes in the margin so that you have a quick reference when you need to review.

Contents

Basic Mathematics Review and Refresher

This unit presents a basic review of Roman numerals, fractions, decimals, and ratio-proportion. Chapter 2 gives an overview of Roman numerals and their Arabic equivalents. The ability to solve for *x* assumes a basic mastery of fractions and decimals. Therefore a brief review of addition, subtraction, multiplication, and division for fractions and decimals has been provided in Chapters 3 and 4 so that you can review this material. In order to accurately calculate dosage problems, you need to be able to transcribe a word problem into a mathematical equation. This process is presented in a "step-by-step" format in Chapter 5. An end-of-unit review is provided for reinforcement of rules.

Preassessment Test: Mathematics Skills Review

Basic math skills are needed to calculate most dosage and solution problems encountered today in clinical practice. This pretest will help you understand your level of competence in solving fraction, decimal, and percentage problems as well as solving for the value of an unknown (*x*) using ratio-proportion.

The pretest has 16 sections comprising 100 questions, each worth one point. Answers are listed in the back of the book. A score of 90% or greater means that you have mastered the knowledge necessary to proceed directly to Unit II. Begin by setting aside 1 hour. You will need scrap paper. Take time to work out your answers and avoid careless mistakes. If an answer is incorrect, please review the corresponding section in Unit I.

Write the following Arabic numbers as Roman numerals.

1. 8 _VIII_ 2. 13 _XIII_

3. 2.5 _iiss_ 4. 37 _XXXVII_

5. 51 _LI_

Write the following Roman numerals as Arabic numbers.

6. xiss __11 1/2__   7. xvi __16__

8. LXV __65__   9. ix __9__

10. XIX __19__

Add or subtract the following fractions. Reduce to lowest terms.

11. $\frac{1}{2} + \frac{1}{8} =$ __5/8__   12. $\frac{3}{4} - \frac{1}{4} =$ __2/4__

13. $\frac{1}{5} + \frac{3}{10} =$ __4/15__   14. $\frac{4}{6} - \frac{2}{5} =$ __2/1__

Choose the fraction that has the largest value.

15. $\frac{1}{3}$ or $\frac{1}{6}$ __1/3__   16. $\frac{1}{150}$ or $\frac{1}{200}$ __1/150__

17. $\frac{1}{100}$ or $\frac{1}{150}$ __1/100__   18. $\frac{1}{2}$ or $\frac{3}{4}$ __3/4__

Multiply or divide the following fractions. Reduce to lowest terms.

19. $\frac{1}{2} \times \frac{3}{4} =$ __3/8__   20. $2\frac{2}{5} \times 3\frac{5}{10}$ __6 10/50 x = 8 2/5__

21. $\frac{1}{4} \div \frac{1}{3} =$ _____   22. $3\frac{1}{2} \div \frac{4}{7} =$ __4/2__

23. $\frac{1}{150} \times 2\frac{1}{2} =$ ____   24. $\frac{8}{7} \times 3 =$ _____

25. $\frac{1}{8} \div 6 =$ _____   26. $4\frac{2}{5} \div 11 =$ _____

Change the following mixed numbers to improper fractions.

27. $2\frac{4}{5}$ _____ 14/5 _____   28. $6\frac{3}{4}$ _____ 27/4 _____

29. $10\frac{4}{9}$ _____ 94/9 _____   30. $8\frac{1}{7}$ _____ 57/7 _____

Reduce these improper fractions to whole or mixed numbers. Reduce to lowest terms.

31. $\frac{120}{40}$ _____ 3 8 _____   32. $\frac{146}{36}$ _____ 2 1 _____

33. $\frac{35}{11}$ _____ 3 _____   34. $\frac{16}{13}$ _____ 1 _____

Change the following fractions to decimals.

35. $\frac{1}{3}$ _____ 0.03 _____   36. $\frac{2}{5}$ _____

37. $\frac{3}{8}$ _____   38. $\frac{3}{4}$ _____ .75 _____

Add or subtract the following decimals.

39. $0.36 + 1.45 =$ _____ 281 1.81 _____

40. $3.71 + 0.29 =$ _____ 4.00 _____

41. $6 - 0.13 =$ _____ 5.87 _____

42. $2.14 - 0.01 =$ _____ 2.13 _____

Multiply or divide the following decimals.

43. $6 \times 8.13 =$ _____ 48.78 _____

44. $0.125 \times 2 =$ _____ 0.25 _____

45. $21.6 \div 0.3 =$ _____

46. $7.82 \div 2.3 =$ _____

Change the following decimals to fractions. Reduce to lowest terms.

47. 0.25 ___1/4___   48. 0.80 _____

49. 0.33 ___1/3___   50. 0.45 _____

51. 0.75 ___3/4___   52. 0.60 _____

Solve for the value of x in the following ratio and proportion problems.

53. $4.2 : 14 :: x : 10$ _____

54. $0.8 : 4 :: 3.2 : x$ _____

55. $6 : 2 :: 8 : x$ _____

56. $5 : 20 :: x : 40$ _____

57. $0.25 : 200 :: x : 600$ _____

58. $\dfrac{1}{5} : x :: \dfrac{1}{20} : 3$ _____

59. $12 : x :: 8 : 16$ _____

60. $x : \dfrac{4}{5} :: 0.60 : 3$ _____

61. $0.3 : 12 :: x : 36$ _____

62. $x : 8 :: \dfrac{1}{4} : 10$ _____

Change the following fractions and decimals to percentages.

63. $\frac{1}{5}$ _____   64. 0.36 _____

65. 0.07 _____   66. $\frac{5}{40}$ _____

67. 0.103 _____   68. 1.83 _____

69. $\frac{4}{16}$ _____   70. 60/100 _____

71. 0.01 _____   72. 1.98 _____

73. $\frac{120}{100}$ _____   74. $\frac{8}{56}$ _____

Change the following percents to decimals.

75. 25% _0.25_   76. 40% _0.40_

77. 80% _0.80_   78. 15% _0.15_

79. 4.8% _0.048_   80. 0.36% _0.036_

81. 1.75% _0.0175_   82. 8.30% _0.0830_

Solve the following percent equations.

83. 30% of 60 _33_

84. 4.5% of 200 _____

85. 0.6% of 180 _____

86. 30 is 75% of _____

87. 20 is 80% of _____

88. What % of 80 is 20 _____

89. What % of 60 is 12 _____

90. What % of 72 is 18 _____

91. 15 is 30% of _____

92. 60 is 50% of _____

Write each of the following measures in its related equivalency. Reduce to lowest terms.

	PERCENT	RATIO	COMMON FRACTION	DECIMAL
93.	25%	_____	_____	_____
94.	_____	1 : 30	_____	_____
95.	_____	_____	_____	0.05
96.	_____	_____	$\frac{1}{150}$	_____
97.	0.45%	_____	_____	_____
98.	_____	1 : 100	_____	_____
99.	_____	_____	$\frac{1}{120}$	_____
100.	_____	_____	_____	0.50

Roman Numerals With Arabic Equivalents

The use of Roman numerals dates back to ancient times when symbols were used for pharmaceutical computations and record keeping. Modern medicine still uses Roman numerals in prescribing medications, especially when using the apothecaries' system of weights and measurement.

The Roman system uses letters to designate numbers; the most commonly used letters can be found in Table 2-1. The most common letters you will use are those between 1/2 (ss̄) and 10 (x). Four numerals are rarely used in practice (50, 100, 500, 1000) but are included in the table for your review.

The Roman numeral system follows certain rules for arrangement of its numerals.

> ► RULE: To read and write Roman
>   numerals, follow these steps:

- ◆ You add values when the *largest* valued numeral is on the *left* and the *smallest* valued numeral is on the *right*.

EXAMPLES: xv = 10 + 5 = 15
             xxv = 20 + 5 = 25

| **TABLE 2-1** |
| Roman Numeral Equivalents for Arabic Numerals |

ARABIC NUMERAL	ROMAN NUMERAL
1/2	ṡ ṡ
1	i
2	ii
3	iii
4	iv
5	v
6	vi
7	vii
8	viii
9	ix
10	x
15	xv
20	xx
30	xxx
50	L
100	C
500	D
1000	M

+ You subtract values when the *smallest* valued numeral is on the *left* and the *largest* valued numeral is on the *right*.

EXAMPLES: ix = 1 − 10 = 9

   iv = 1 − 5 = 4

+ You *subtract* values *first* and then *add* when the *smallest* valued numeral is in the *middle* and the *larger* values are on either side.

EXAMPLES: xiv = (1 − 5) = 4 + 10 = 14

   xix = (1 − 10) = 9 + 10 = 19

> ► RULE: To repeat Roman numerals, follow this step:

+ Roman numerals of the same value can be repeated in sequence, *only up to three times.* Once you can no longer repeat, you need to subtract.

EXAMPLES: 3 = iii

   4 = 5 (v) − 1 (i) = iv

   9 = 10 (x) − 1 (i) = ix

   30 = 10 (x) + 10 (x) + 10 (x) = xxx

   40 = 50 (L) − 10 (X) = XL

Note: Three numerals *may never be repeated* in sequence because their values, when doubled, become separate Roman numerals. These are L, V, and D.

EXAMPLES: X   10   not   VV

             C   100   not   LL

             M   1000   not   DD

➤ *PRACTICE PROBLEMS* ➤

Change the following Arabic numerals to Roman numerals:

1. $\frac{1}{2}$ _____ ss   2. 3 _____ III

3. 7 _____ VII   4. 10 _____ X

5. 15 _____ XVi   6. 30 _____ XXX

Change the following Roman numerals to Arabic numerals:

7. vi _____ L   8. ii _____ 2

9. v _____ 5   10. ix _____ 9

11. xx _____ 20   12. xxv _____ 25

END OF CHAPTER REVIEW

Write the following Arabic numerals as Roman numerals:

1. 27 _____ XXVII   2. 32 _____ XXXII

3. 16 _____ XVI   4. 4 _____ IIII IV

5. 8 _VIII_ 6. 10 _X_

7. 12 _XII_ 8. 21 _XXI_

9. 18 _~~XIII IIXX~~ XVIII_ 10. 24 _XXIV_

Write the following Roman numerals as Arabic numerals:

11. xviii _18_ 12. xvi _16_

13. ss _1/2_ 14. ix _9_

15. vii ss _7 1/2_ 16. xix _19_

17. xxiv _24_ 18. xiv _14_

19. xxvi _26_ 20. vi _6_

3

Common Fractions

Many drug preparations are prescribed and prepared in fractions. You will need to know how to calculate drug dosages when fractions are used.

A *fraction* is a portion or piece of a whole that indicates division of that whole into equal units or parts. If you divide an apple into four equal parts, the *total number of parts* (4) that you are working with is the *bottom* number of the fraction and is called the *denominator*. Each part or fraction of the apple that is considered (1) is the *top* number of the fraction and is called the *numerator*.

Look at the example below:

$$\text{Fraction} = \frac{1}{4} = \frac{\text{numerator}}{\text{denominator}}$$

For the fraction $\frac{1}{4}$, 1 is the numerator, and 4 is the denominator.

Remember the following rule:

> ▶ RULE: The numerator refers to a *part* of the whole and is the number on the top of the fraction. The denominator refers to the *total number* of parts and is the number on the bottom of the fraction.

➤ *PRACTICE PROBLEMS* ➤

For the following fractions, place an "N" next to the numerator and a "D" next to the denominator.

1. $\frac{4}{5}$ ⁿ ᴅ _____

2. $\frac{1}{2}$ N/D _____

3. $\frac{3}{8}$ ⁿ ᴅ _____

4. $\frac{4}{9}$ N/D _____

5. $\frac{7}{8}$ ⁿ ᴅ _____

6. $\frac{1}{6}$ ᴜ ᴅ _____

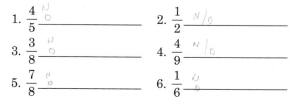

⊕ THE NUMERATOR OF A FRACTION

The numerator tells you how many equal parts you have. For example, the numerator 2 in the fraction 2/3 tells you that you have *two* equal parts of three that are each worth 1/3. The numerator 3 in the fraction 3/5 tells you that you have *three* equal parts of five that are each worth 1/5.

➤ *PRACTICE PROBLEMS* ➤

Look at the following first example problem below. Then fill in the blanks for the rest.

1. 7/8 means that you have __7__ equal parts worth __1/8__ each.

2. 9/10 means that you have __9__ equal parts worth __1/10__ each.

3. 4/5 means that you have __4__ equal parts worth __1/5__ each.

4. 3/4 means that you have __3__ equal parts worth __1/4__ each.

5. 2/7 means that you have __2__ equal parts
   worth __1/7__ each.

THE DENOMINATOR OF A FRACTION

The denominator of a fraction tells you the total number of equal parts into which the whole has been divided. For example, if you divide something into four equal parts, each part would be expressed as a fraction that has the denominator of 4. That is, each part would be equal to 1/4. If you divide something into eight equal parts, the denominator would be 8, and each part would be equal to 1/8. Look at Figure 3-1, which illustrates two circles: one is divided into fourths, and one is divided into eighths.

As you look at the circles, you will notice that the circle that is divided into eighths has smaller portions than the circle that is divided into fourths. The reason is that the value of each part of the fraction 1/8 is less than the value of each part of the fraction 1/4. Even though 1/8 has a larger denominator (8) than does 1/4 (4), it is a smaller fraction. This is an important concept to understand, that is, the larger the number or value in the denominator, the smaller the fraction or pieces of the whole. To clarify, consider these examples:

$$\frac{1}{2} \text{ is larger than } \frac{1}{4}$$

$$\frac{1}{8} \text{ is larger than } \frac{1}{16}$$

$$\frac{1}{9} \text{ is larger than } \frac{1}{10}$$

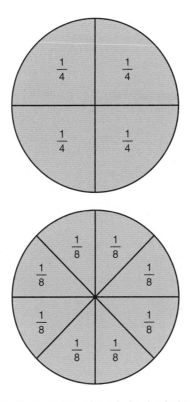

Figure 3-1. Two circles: The whole divided into equal parts.

Remember the following rule:

> ► RULE: The larger the number in the denominator, the smaller the value of the pieces (or fraction) of the whole.

➤ *PRACTICE PROBLEMS* ➤

Arrange the following fractions in order of size. That is, list the fraction with the *smallest value first,* then the next larger fraction, and so on until you end with the *largest valued fraction last.*

$$\frac{1}{9} \quad \frac{1}{12} \quad \frac{1}{3} \quad \frac{1}{7} \quad \frac{1}{150} \quad \frac{1}{25} \quad \frac{1}{100} \quad \frac{1}{300} \quad \frac{1}{75}$$

¹/₃₀₀ ¹/₁₅₀ ¹/₁₀₀ ¹/₇₅ ¹/₂₅ ¹/₁₂ ¹/₉ ¹/₇ ¹/₃

✦ FRACTIONS THAT ARE LESS THAN ONE, EQUAL TO ONE, OR MORE THAN ONE

The following rules tell you how to decide if a fraction is less than one (< 1), equal to one, or more than one (> 1).

> ➤ RULE: If the numerator is less than the denominator, the fraction value is *less than* one. These fractions are called *proper* fractions.

EXAMPLES: $\frac{3}{4} < 1, \quad \frac{7}{8} < 1, \quad \frac{9}{10} < 1$

> ➤ RULE: If the numerator and denominator are equal to each other, the fraction value is equal to one. These fractions are called *improper* fractions.

EXAMPLES: $\dfrac{1}{1} = 1, \quad \dfrac{3}{3} = 1, \quad \dfrac{25}{25} = 1$

> ► RULE: If the numerator is *greater than* the denominator, the fraction value is more than one. These fractions are also called *improper* fractions.

EXAMPLES: $\dfrac{2}{1} = 2 > 1, \quad \dfrac{5}{4} = 1\dfrac{1}{4} > 1$

✛ MIXED NUMBERS AND IMPROPER FRACTIONS

To calculate drug dosages, you need to know how to convert fractions and reduce them to their lowest terms. Following are some common rules.

> ► RULE: If a fraction and a whole number are *written together*, the fraction value is *more than one*. These fractions are called *mixed* numbers.

EXAMPLES: $1\dfrac{1}{2}, \quad 3\dfrac{3}{4}, \quad 5\dfrac{4}{5}$

Mixed numbers can be changed to improper fractions. For example, 1 1/2 can be changed to 3/2. The following rule tells you how to change a mixed number to an improper fraction.

Changing a Mixed Number to an Improper Fraction

> ➤ RULE: To change a mixed number to an improper fraction, follow these steps:

- ◆ Multiply the denominator by the whole number. That is, if you have the fraction of 2 3/4, you would multiply 4 × 2, which equals 8.
- ◆ Add the numerator (3) to the answer you got when you multiplied the denominator by the whole number (8) in the preceding step. Using the previous example, this means that you would add 3 to 8 and get the answer of 11.
- ◆ The answer that you got (11) becomes the new numerator of the new single fraction. The denominator in the original mixed fraction (which is 4 in this example) stays the same.

The *mixed number* 2 3/4 becomes the *improper fraction* 11/4.

➤ PRACTICE PROBLEMS ➤

Change the following mixed numbers to improper fractions:

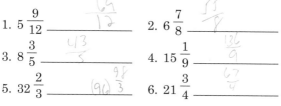

1. $5 \dfrac{9}{12}$ _____   2. $6 \dfrac{7}{8}$ _____

3. $8 \dfrac{3}{5}$ _____   4. $15 \dfrac{1}{9}$ _____

5. $32 \dfrac{2}{3}$ _____   6. $21 \dfrac{3}{4}$ _____

7. $18\frac{1}{2}$ _____

8. $6\frac{3}{9}$ _____

9. $5\frac{2}{5}$ _____

10. $11\frac{1}{6}$ _____

Improper fractions can also be changed to mixed numbers or a whole number. For example, the fraction 5/4 can be changed to 1 1/4. Often when you are working the mathematics for a given problem, you will need to work with improper fractions. However, if you get a final answer that is an improper fraction, convert it to a mixed number. For example, it is better to say "I have 1 1/4 apples" than to say "I have 5/4 apples."

Look at the following rule, which tells you how to change an improper fraction to a mixed number.

Changing an Improper Fraction to a Mixed Number

> ▶ RULE: To change an improper fraction to a mixed number, follow these steps:

♦ The numerator is divided by the denominator. If you use the example of 13/7, this means you would divide 13 by 7:

$$7\overline{)13} \atop \frac{1}{}$$

$$\frac{7}{6} \text{ left over}$$

- The number that you get when you divide the numerator by the denominator becomes the whole number of the mixed number. In the preceding example, (1) becomes the whole number.
- The *remainder,* or number that you have left over (6 in the previous example), becomes the numerator of the fraction that goes with the whole number to make it a mixed number. Using the preceding example, your answer would look like this so far: 1 6/?.
- The *original* denominator of the fraction of the mixed number (which is 7 in this case) becomes the denominator of the fraction of the mixed number. In this example, the improper fraction 13/7 becomes the mixed number 1 6/7.
- Any remainder is reduced to the lowest terms.

> ➤ PRACTICE PROBLEMS ➤

Change the following improper fractions to mixed numbers:

1. $\dfrac{30}{4}$ _____

2. $\dfrac{41}{6}$ _____

3. $\dfrac{68}{9}$ _____

4. $\dfrac{72}{11}$ _____

5. $\dfrac{90}{12}$ _____

6. $\dfrac{40}{15}$ _____

7. $\dfrac{86}{20}$ _____

8. $\dfrac{62}{8}$ _____

9. $\dfrac{86}{9}$ _____

10. $\dfrac{112}{6}$ _____

⊕ EQUIVALENT OR EQUAL FRACTIONS

Changing Fractions to Equivalent or Equal Fractions

When you are working problems with fractions, it is sometimes necessary to change a fraction to a different but equivalent fraction. For example, it may be necessary to change 2/4 to 1/2 or 2/3 to 4/6. You can make a new fraction that has the same value by either multiplying or dividing *both* the numerator and the denominator by the *same* number. Look at the following examples.

EXAMPLES: $\frac{2}{3}$ can be changed to $\frac{4}{6}$ by multiplying both the numerator and the denominator by 2.

$$\left(\frac{2}{3} \times \frac{2}{2} = \frac{4}{6}\right)$$

$\frac{2}{4}$ can be changed to $\frac{1}{2}$ by dividing both the numerator and the denominator by 2.

$$\left(\frac{2}{4} \div \frac{2}{2} = \frac{1}{2}\right)$$

It is important to remember that you can change the numerator and the denominator of a fraction and still keep the same value *so long as you follow the following rule:*

> ▶ RULE: When changing a fraction, you
> must do the same thing (multiply or
> divide by the same number) to the
> numerator and to the denominator in
> order to keep the same value.

EXAMPLES: To change the fraction $\frac{4}{5}$ to $\frac{8}{10}$, multiply 4×2 and 5×2.

$$\left(\frac{4 \times 2 = 8}{5 \times 2 = 10} \right)$$

$\frac{4}{5}$ has the same value as $\frac{8}{10}$.

To change the fraction $\frac{4}{16}$ to $\frac{1}{4}$, divide 4 by 4 and 16 by 4.

$$\left(\frac{4 \div 4 = 1}{16 \div 4 = 4} \right)$$

To determine that both fractions have equal value, multiply the opposite numerators and denominators. For example, if 4/5 = 8/10, then the product of 4×10 will equal the product of 5×8.

$$4 \times 10 = 40 \text{ and } 5 \times 8 = 40$$

➤ *PRACTICE PROBLEMS* ➤

1. 3/5 is equivalent to: 6/15 or 9/10 or 12/20

2. 4/8 is equivalent to: 8/24 or 12/16 or 20/40

    _____

3. 6/12 is equivalent to: 2/4 or 3/5 or 12/36

    _____

4. 10/16 is equivalent to: 20/48 or 5/8 or 30/32

    _____

5. 12/20 is equivalent to: 3/5 or 6/5 or 4/10

    _____

6. 18/30 is equivalent to: 3/15 or 9/10 or 6/10

    _____

7. 9/54 is equivalent to: 3/16 or 1/6 or 1/8

    _____

8. 15/90 is equivalent to: 1/6 or 3/8 or 5/14

    _____

9. 14/56 is equivalent to: 2/6 or 1/4 or 7/8

    _____

10. 8/144 is equivalent to: 2/36 or 4/23 or 1/18

    _____

⊕ SIMPLIFYING, OR REDUCING, FRACTIONS

When calculating dosages, it is easier to work with fractions that have been simplified, or reduced to the lowest terms. This means that the numerator and the denominator are the smallest numbers that can still represent the fraction or piece of the whole. For example, 4/10 can be reduced to 2/5; 4/8 can be reduced to 1/2. It is important to know how to reduce (or simplify) a fraction. The following rule outlines the steps for reducing a fraction to the lowest terms:

> ➤ RULE: To reduce a fraction to its lowest terms, follow these steps:

- Study both the numerator and the denominator and determine the largest number that can go evenly into *both* the numerator *and* the denominator. For example, suppose you were trying to reduce the fraction 9/18. The largest number that will go into *both* the numerator (9) and the denominator (18) is 9.
- Divide *both* the numerator and the denominator by the number that you determined will go evenly into both of them. Using the preceding example, this means you would do the following:

$$\left(\frac{9 \ \div \ 9 \ = \ 1}{18 \ \div \ 9 \ = \ 2} \right)$$

Consider these examples:

$\frac{6}{10}$ can be reduced to $\frac{3}{5}$ by dividing both the numerator and the denominator by 2.

$\frac{5}{15}$ can be reduced to $\frac{1}{3}$ by dividing both the numerator and the denominator by 5.

➤ *PRACTICE PROBLEMS* ➤

Reduce the following fractions to their lowest terms:

1. $\frac{8}{48}$ —————————— 2. $\frac{6}{36}$ ——————————

3. $\frac{4}{36}$ ——————————

⊕ ADDITION OF FRACTIONS

Fractions can be added only when the denominators are the same because only the numerators are added. Unlike denominators must be made similar.

Addition of Fractions With Like Denominators

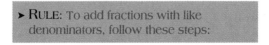

> ➤ RULE: To add fractions with like denominators, follow these steps:

- Add the numerators. For example, to add 1/5 + 3/5, add the numerators 1 + 3 = 4.

- Place the new sum over the like denominator that remains the same. Place 4 over 5 or 4/5.
- Reduce to lowest terms, if necessary.
- Change any improper fraction to a mixed number.

EXAMPLES: $\dfrac{1}{7} + \dfrac{4}{7}$

Change: $\dfrac{1}{7} + \dfrac{4}{7} = \dfrac{1}{7} + \dfrac{4}{7} = \dfrac{5}{7}$

5 = new numerator

7 = like denominator

$Answer = \dfrac{5}{7}$

EXAMPLES: $\dfrac{1}{6} + \dfrac{9}{6}$

Change: $\dfrac{1}{6} + \dfrac{9}{6} = \dfrac{1}{6} + \dfrac{9}{6} = \dfrac{10}{6}$

10 = new numerator

6 = like denominator

$\dfrac{10}{6}$ needs to be reduced

Reduce:

$\dfrac{10}{6} = \dfrac{10 \div 2}{6 \div 2} = \dfrac{5}{3} = $ improper fraction

Change: $\dfrac{5}{3} = 5 \div 3 = 1\dfrac{2}{3}$

$Answer = 1\dfrac{2}{3}$

Addition of Fractions With Unlike Denominators

> ► RULE: To add fractions with unlike denominators, follow these steps:

- ◆ Find the least common denominator. The *easiest* way to find the least common denominator is to find the lowest number that is easily divisible by both denominators. For example, to add 1/4 + 3/5, use the least common denominator of 20.
- ◆ Change the unlike fractions to like fractions.

1. Divide the common denominator of 20 by the denominator of each fraction.

$$\text{For the fraction } \frac{1}{4},$$

$$\text{divide } 4\overline{)20} \quad \overset{5 \text{ (quotient)}}{}$$

$$\text{For the fraction } \frac{3}{5},$$

$$\text{divide } 5\overline{)20} \quad \overset{4 \text{ (quotient)}}{}$$

2. Take each new quotient and multiply it by the numerator of each fraction.

For the fraction 1/4, multiply the numerator 1 by the quotient 5 for the new numerator of 5.

For the fraction 3/5, multiply the numerator 3 by the quotient 4 for a new numerator of 12.

$$\frac{1}{4} \text{ becomes } \frac{5}{20}$$

$$\frac{3}{5} \text{ becomes } \frac{12}{20}$$

• Add the new numerators and place your answer over the common denominator. Reduce to lowest terms, if necessary.

$$5 + 12 = 17$$

$$Answer = \frac{17}{20}$$

EXAMPLE: Add $\frac{1}{3} + \frac{5}{6}$

A common denominator would be 18 (6 × 3).

Change $\frac{1}{3}$ to $\frac{6}{18}$

Change $\frac{5}{6}$ to $\frac{15}{18}$

Add the new numerators.

$6 + 15 = \frac{21}{18}$ needs to be reduced to $\frac{7}{6}$

$\frac{7}{6}$ should be changed to $1\frac{1}{6}$

$$Answer = 1\frac{1}{6}$$

✛ ADDITION OF MIXED NUMBERS

> ► RULE: To add fractions with a mixed number, follow these steps:

- Change the mixed number to an improper fraction.
  To add 1/6 + 2 3/8 + 5/6, change 2 3/8 to 19/8.
- Find the least common denominator. For the denominators of 6 and 8, use the least common denominator of 24.
- Change the unlike fractions to like fractions.

$$\frac{1}{6} \text{ becomes } \frac{4}{24}$$

$$\frac{19}{8} \text{ becomes } \frac{57}{24}$$

$$\frac{5}{6} \text{ becomes } \frac{20}{24}$$

- Add the new numerators and place your answer over the common denominator.

$$4 + 57 + 20 = \frac{81}{24}$$

- Reduce, if necessary.

$$\frac{81}{24} = \frac{27}{8} = 3\frac{3}{8}$$

Answer $= 3\frac{3}{8}$

⊕ SUBTRACTION OF FRACTIONS

Fractions can be subtracted only when the denominators are the same because only the numerators are subtracted. Unlike denominators must be made similar.

Subtraction of Fractions with Like Denominators

> ► RULE: To subtract fractions with like denominators, subtract the numerators.

To subtract fractions with like denominators, simply subtract the numerators. If you need to subtract 3/8 from 7/8, simply subtract 3 from 7, which equals 4. Place the new numerator 4 over 8 and reduce to its lowest terms (1/2).

EXAMPLES:
$$\frac{5}{6} - \frac{3}{6} = 5 - 3 = 2$$

$$\frac{2}{6} = \frac{1}{3}, \text{ a new fraction}$$

$$\frac{7}{8} - \frac{4}{8} = 7 - 4 = 3$$

$$\frac{3}{8}, \text{ a new fraction}$$

Subtraction of Fractions with Unlike Denominators

You will probably never need to subtract unlike fractions or fractions with a mixed number to calculate dosage problems. However, both will be presented here briefly in case you want to review the steps.

> ► RULE: To subtract fractions with unlike denominators, follow these steps:

- ◆ Find the least common denominator. To subtract 3/5 from 5/6, use the least common denominator of 30.
- ◆ Change the unlike fractions to like fractions. (Refer to pages 23–24 to review changing unlike fractions to like fractions if you need help.)

$$\frac{5}{6} \text{ becomes } \frac{25}{30}$$

$$\frac{3}{5} \text{ becomes } \frac{18}{30}$$

- ◆ Subtract the new numerators and place your answer over the common denominator: $25 - 18 = 7$, the new numerator. Place 7 over 30, 7/30.

$$Answer = \frac{7}{30}$$

Subtraction of Mixed Numbers

There are two methods of subtracting mixed numbers:

1. Subtract the fractions by changing the mixed number to an improper fraction. For example,

to subtract 3/6 from 2 1/8, you want to change
the mixed number (2 1/8) to an improper
fraction.

> ► RULE: To subtract fractions with a mixed
> number, follow these steps:

♦ Change the mixed number to an improper
  fraction.

  To subtract 3/6 from 2 1/8, change 2 1/8 to
  17/8.

♦ Find the least common denominator. For the
  denominators 8 and 6, use the least common
  denominator of 24.

♦ Change the unlike fractions to like fractions.

$$\frac{17}{8} \text{ becomes } \frac{51}{24}$$

$$\frac{3}{6} \text{ becomes } \frac{12}{24}$$

♦ Subtract the new numerators and place your
  answer over the common denominator: $51 -
  12 = 39$, the new numerator.

$$\frac{39}{24} \text{ becomes } \frac{13}{8} = 1\frac{5}{8}$$

$$Answer = 1\frac{5}{8}$$

2. Subtract the fractions by leaving the mixed
   number as is. For example, to subtract 3/6
   from 2 1/8 you can leave 2 1/8 as is and set up
   your subtraction like this:

$$2\frac{1}{8}$$

$$-\frac{3}{6}$$

> **RULE:** To subtract fractions with a mixed number, follow these steps:

- Find the least common denominator. For the denominators of 6 and 8, use the least common denominator of 24.
- Change the unlike denominators.

$$2\frac{1}{8} \text{ becomes } 2\frac{3}{24}$$

$$\frac{3}{6} \text{ becomes } \frac{12}{24}$$

- Subtract the numerators; subtract the whole numbers.

Note: To subtract 12/24 from 2 3/24 you need to borrow 1 or 24/24 from the whole number 2. Add 24 to 3 = 27, a new numerator.

EXAMPLE:

$$2\frac{3}{24} = 1\frac{27}{24}$$

$$-\frac{12}{24} = -\frac{12}{24}$$

$$\overline{\phantom{-\frac{12}{24}}}\qquad \overline{1\frac{15}{24}} = 1\frac{5}{8}$$

$$\textit{Answer} = 1\frac{5}{8}$$

➤ PRACTICE PROBLEMS ➤

Addition of Fractions

1. $\dfrac{5}{11} + \dfrac{9}{11} + \dfrac{13}{11} =$ _____

2. $\dfrac{7}{16} + \dfrac{3}{8} =$ _____

3. $\dfrac{4}{6} + 3\dfrac{1}{8} =$ _____

4. $\dfrac{11}{15} + \dfrac{14}{45} =$ _____

5. $\dfrac{5}{20} + \dfrac{8}{20} + \dfrac{13}{20} =$ _____

Subtraction of Fractions

6. $\dfrac{6}{7} - \dfrac{3}{7} =$ _____   7. $\dfrac{8}{9} - \dfrac{4}{9} =$ _____

8. $\dfrac{3}{5} - \dfrac{1}{6} =$ _____   9. $\dfrac{3}{4} - \dfrac{2}{9} =$ _____

10. $6\dfrac{3}{7} - \dfrac{2}{3} =$ _____

✛ MULTIPLICATION OF FRACTIONS

Multiplying a Fraction by Another Fraction

Multiplying fractions is easy. All that you have to do is multiply the numerators by each other, and the denominators by each other. For example, if you want to multiply 3/4 by 2/3, you would multiply 3×2, to get the new numerator, and 4×3, to get the new denominator.

> ► RULE: To multiply fractions, multiply the numerators to get the new numerator, and multiply the denominators to get the new denominator. Reduce the product to its lowest terms.

EXAMPLE: $\dfrac{3}{4} \times \dfrac{2}{3} = \dfrac{6}{12}$ or $\dfrac{1}{2}$ $\dfrac{1}{2} \times \dfrac{2}{3} = \dfrac{2}{6}$ or $\dfrac{1}{3}$

This method of multiplying fractions is sometimes considered to be the "long form" or long method. There is also a "shortcut" method for multiplying fractions, called "cancellation." With cancellation, you actually simplify the numbers *before* you multiply by reducing the numbers to their lowest terms. Look at the example below:

EXAMPLE: $\dfrac{1}{4} \times \dfrac{8}{15}$

Cancellation can be used because the denominator of the first fraction (4) and the numerator of the second fraction (8) can both be divided by 4 and the value of the fraction does not change. So, if you work the problem, it looks like this:

$$\dfrac{1}{4} \times \dfrac{8}{15} = \dfrac{1}{4_1} \times \dfrac{8^2}{15}$$

Once you have canceled all the numbers and reduced them to the lowest terms, you can then multiply the new numerators and the new denominators to get your answer.

$$\dfrac{1}{1} \times \dfrac{2}{15} = \dfrac{2}{15}$$

Answer $= \dfrac{2}{15}$

Multiplying a Fraction by a Mixed Number

Whenever you have to multiply a mixed number, you should always convert it to an improper fraction before you work the problem. Remember the following rule:

> ► RULE: To multiply a fraction that involves a mixed number, change the mixed number to an improper fraction before you work the problem.

EXAMPLES: $1\frac{1}{2} \times \frac{1}{2}$

Change: $1\frac{1}{2}$ to $\frac{3}{2}$

Multiply: $\frac{3}{2} \times \frac{1}{2} = \frac{3}{4}$

$$Answer = \frac{3}{4}$$

$1\frac{1}{2} \times 4\frac{1}{2}$

Change: $1\frac{1}{2}$ to $\frac{3}{2}$

Change: $4\frac{1}{2}$ to $\frac{9}{2}$

Multiply: $\frac{3}{2} \times \frac{9}{2} = \frac{27}{4}$ or $6\frac{3}{4}$

$$Answer = 6\frac{3}{4}$$

⊕ DIVISION OF FRACTIONS

Dividing a Fraction by Another Fraction

Sometimes it is necessary to divide fractions in order to calculate a drug dosage.

> ▶ RULE: To divide fractions, follow these steps:

• Write your problem.

EXAMPLE: $\dfrac{4}{5} \div \dfrac{5}{9}$

• Invert the divisor, the number by which you are dividing. This means that 5/9 becomes 9/5.
• Multiply your fractions and reduce them to the lowest terms. If you use the preceding example, your problem now looks like this:

$$\frac{4}{5} \times \frac{9}{5} = \frac{36}{25} = 1\frac{11}{25}$$

$$Answer = 1\frac{11}{25}$$

EXAMPLE: $\dfrac{7}{8} \div \dfrac{3}{5}$

Invert: $\dfrac{3}{5}$ to $\dfrac{5}{3}$

Multiply: $\dfrac{7}{8} \times \dfrac{5}{3} = \dfrac{35}{24} = 1\dfrac{11}{24}$

$$Answer = 1\frac{11}{24}$$

Dividing a Fraction by a Mixed Number

To divide a mixed number, always convert the mixed number to an improper fraction before you work your problem.

> ▶ RULE: To divide a fraction that involves a mixed number, change the mixed number to an improper fraction and reduce to the lowest terms.

EXAMPLE: $\dfrac{3}{6} \div 1\dfrac{2}{5}$

Change: $1\dfrac{2}{5}$ to $\dfrac{7}{5}$

Write: $\dfrac{3}{6} \div \dfrac{7}{5}$

Invert: $\dfrac{7}{5}$ to $\dfrac{5}{7}$

Multiply: $\dfrac{3}{6} \times \dfrac{5}{7} = \dfrac{15}{42} = \dfrac{5}{14}$

$$Answer = \dfrac{5}{14}$$

➤ PRACTICE PROBLEMS ➤

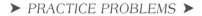

Multiplication of Fractions

1. $\dfrac{7}{15} \times \dfrac{8}{12} =$ _____   2. $\dfrac{5}{9} \times \dfrac{3}{7} =$ _____

3. $\dfrac{6}{16} \times \dfrac{2}{5} =$ _____   4. $2\dfrac{7}{10} \times \dfrac{1}{2} =$ _____

5. $3\frac{4}{8} \times \frac{3}{16} =$ _____

Division of Fractions

6. $\frac{3}{4} \div \frac{1}{9} =$ _____   7. $\frac{6}{13} \div \frac{2}{5} =$ _____

8. $\frac{8}{12} \div \frac{3}{7} =$ _____   9. $12 \div \frac{1}{3} =$ _____

10. $8\frac{7}{10} \div 15 =$ _____

END OF CHAPTER REVIEW

Change the unlike fractions to like fractions by find-ing a common denominator:

1. $\frac{2}{5}, \frac{3}{7}$ _____   2. $\frac{7}{5}, \frac{4}{20}$ _____

Reduce the following fractions to their lowest terms:

3. $\frac{27}{162}$ _____   4. $\frac{16}{128}$ _____

Change the following improper fractions to mixed numbers:

5. $\frac{26}{4}$ _____   6. $\frac{105}{8}$ _____

Change the following mixed numbers to improper fractions:

7. $4\frac{6}{11}$ _____   8. $9\frac{2}{23}$ _____

Reduce the following fractions to their lowest terms:

9. $\dfrac{20}{64}$ _____   10. $\dfrac{16}{128}$ _____

11. $\dfrac{7}{63}$ _____

Add the following fractions:

12. $\dfrac{1}{9} + \dfrac{7}{9} =$ _____   13. $\dfrac{5}{6} + \dfrac{3}{6} =$ _____

14. $\dfrac{1}{9} + \dfrac{3}{4} =$ _____   15. $6\dfrac{5}{6} + \dfrac{3}{8} =$ _____

Subtract the following fractions:

16. $\dfrac{5}{12} - \dfrac{3}{12} =$ _____   17. $\dfrac{7}{9} - \dfrac{2}{9} =$ _____

18. $\dfrac{3}{4} - \dfrac{1}{6} =$ _____   19. $4\dfrac{6}{10} - \dfrac{3}{8} =$ _____

20. $6\dfrac{3}{8} - 4\dfrac{1}{4} =$ _____

Multiply the following fractions:

21. $\dfrac{6}{8} \times \dfrac{1}{5} =$ _____   22. $\dfrac{9}{11} \times \dfrac{1}{3} =$ _____

23. $2\dfrac{1}{10} \times 6\dfrac{6}{9} =$ _____   24. $2\dfrac{2}{7} \times 3\dfrac{4}{8} =$ _____

25. $1\dfrac{5}{11} \times \dfrac{3}{8} =$ _____

Divide the following fractions:

26. $\dfrac{3}{5} \div \dfrac{7}{20} =$ _____   27. $\dfrac{8}{9} \div \dfrac{1}{27} =$ _____

28. $6\dfrac{5}{12} \div \dfrac{15}{24} =$ _____   29. $7\dfrac{2}{14} \div 80 =$ _____

20. $16 \div \dfrac{32}{160} =$ _____

Decimals or Decimal Fractions

Medications are frequently prescribed in decimals, and you will find that many of your dosage problems will be worked out using the decimal format. A decimal indicates the "tenths" of a number because a decimal is a fraction with a denominator of any multiple of 10. A decimal's value is determined by its position to the right of a decimal point. Always add a zero (0) to the left of the decimal point to avoid errors in reading the value. In other words:

0.2 is read as 2 tenths because the number 2 is one position to the right of the decimal point.

0.03 is read as 3 hundredths because the number 3 is two positions to the right of the decimal point.

0.004 is read as 4 thousandths because the number 4 is three positions to the right of the decimal point.

0.150 is read as 15 hundredths because the zero after the 15 does not enhance its value.

Whole Numbers	↑
Ten thousands	10,000
Thousands (Kilo)	1000
Hundreds (Hecto)	100
Tens (Deka)	10
Ones	1
Decimal Point	
Tenths (Deci)	.1
Hundredths (Centi)	.01
Thousandths (Milli)	.001
Ten thousandths	.0001
Hundred thousandths	.00001
Decimal Numbers	↓

Figure 4-1. Numbers read according to their decimal place value. Prefixes describe decimal value.

Figure 4-1 may help you understand a decimal's position. Moving quickly up and down the scale can occur simply by moving the decimal to the left or right as explained on pages 51–53.

When reading a decimal, it is important to remember that numbers to the right of the decimal point have a value *less than 1* and numbers to the left of the decimal point have a value *greater than 1*. Remember the following rule:

> ➤ RULE: Numbers to the right of the decimal point have a value less than 1, and numbers to the left of the decimal point have a value greater than 1.

To read a decimal fraction, follow these steps:

- Read figures to the left of the decimal point as whole numbers.
- Read the decimal point as "and" or "point."
- Read the decimal number to the right of the decimal point as the fraction.

EXAMPLES:

Read:

5	.	2		6	.	0 3	0 . 0 0 4
five	and	two tenths		six	and	three hundredths	four thousandths

➤ *PRACTICE PROBLEMS* ➤

Write the following decimals as you would read them:

1. 10.001 _____

2. 3.0007 _____

3. 0.083 _____

4. 0.153 _____

5. 36.0067 _____

6. 0.0125 _____

7. 125.025 _____

8. 20.075 _____

Write the following decimals:

9. Five and thirty-seven thousandths

    _____

10. Sixty-four and seven hundredths

    _____

11. Twenty thousandths

    _____

12. Four tenths

    _____

13. Eight and sixty-four thousandths

    _____

14. Thirty-three and seven tenths

    _____

15. Fifteen thousandths

    _____

16. One tenth

    _____

⊕ ADDITION OF DECIMALS

> ➤ RULE: To add decimals, follow these
> steps:

- Place the decimals to be added in a vertical
  column with the decimal points directly
  under one another. Add zeros to balance the
  columns if necessary. If you want to add 0.5,
  3.24, and 8, then you would place the
  numbers like this:

$$
\begin{array}{r}
0.50 \\
3.24 \\
+\ 8.00 \\
\end{array}
$$

- Add the decimals in the same manner as
  whole numbers are added.

$$
\begin{array}{r}
0.50 \\
3.24 \\
+\ 8.00 \\
\hline
11.74 \\
\end{array}
$$

- Place the decimal in the answer directly
  under aligned decimal points.

EXAMPLES: 3.9 + 4.7

$$
\begin{array}{r}
3.9 \\
+\ 4.7 \\
\hline
8.6 \\
\end{array}
$$

Answer = 8.6

$$6 + 2.8 + 1.6$$

$$\begin{array}{r} 6.0 \\ 2.8 \\ + 1.6 \\ \hline 10.4 \end{array}$$

Answer = 10.4

SUBTRACTION OF DECIMALS

> ➤ RULE: To subtract decimals, follow these steps:

♦ Place the decimals to be subtracted in a vertical column with the decimal points directly under one another. Add zeros to balance the columns if necessary. If you want to subtract 4.1 from 6.2, you would place the numbers like this:

$$\begin{array}{r} 6.2 \\ - 4.1 \\ \hline \end{array}$$

♦ Subtract the decimals in the same manner as whole numbers as subtracted.

$$\begin{array}{r} 6.2 \\ - 4.1 \\ \hline 2.1 \end{array}$$

- Place the decimal point in the answer directly under the aligned decimal points.

EXAMPLES: 16.84 − 1.32

$$\begin{array}{r} 16.84 \\ -\ 1.32 \\ \hline 15.52 \end{array}$$

Answer = 15.52

13.60 − 8.00

$$\begin{array}{r} 13.60 \\ -\ 8.00 \\ \hline 5.60 \end{array}$$

Answer = 5.60

7.02 − 3.0086

$$\begin{array}{r} 7.0200 \\ -\ 3.0086 \\ \hline 4.0114 \end{array}$$

Answer = 4.0114

✇ MULTIPLICATION OF DECIMALS

Multiplication of Decimal Numbers

Multiplication of decimals is done using the same method as is used for multiplying whole numbers. The major concern is placement of the decimal point in the product.

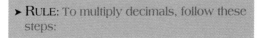

> ➤ RULE: To multiply decimals, follow these steps:

- Place the decimals to be multiplied in the same position as whole numbers would be placed. If you want to multiply 6.3 by 7.6, then place the numbers like this:

$$\begin{array}{r} 6.3 \\ \times\ 7.6 \end{array}$$

- Multiply the decimal numbers as you would multiply whole numbers. Write down the product without the decimal point.

$$\begin{array}{r} 6.3 \\ \times\ 7.6 \\ \hline 378 \\ 441\ \ \\ \hline 4788 \end{array} \text{ product}$$

- Count off the number of decimal places *to the right* of the decimals in the two numbers being multiplied. Then count off the total number of places in the product. For example:

$$\begin{array}{r} 6.3 \\ \times\ 7.6 \\ \hline 378 \\ 441\ \ \\ \hline 47.88 \end{array}$$

   6.3   one place to right of decimal
× 7.6   + one place to right of decimal
  378
441
47.88   two places, count off right to left
   ↑⎵

Answer = 47.88

⊕ MULTIPLICATION BY 10, 100, OR 1000

Multiplying by 10, 100, or 1000 is a fast and easy way to calculate dosage problems. Simply move the decimal point the same number of places to the right as there are zeros in the multiplier. See Table 4-1.

EXAMPLE: 0.712×10. There is one zero in the multiplier of ten. Move the decimal one place to the right for an answer of 7.12.

$$0.712 = 0.712 = 7.12$$

EXAMPLE: 0.08×1000. There are three zeros in the multiplier of 1000. Move the decimal three places to the right for an answer of 80.

$$0.08 = 0.080 = 80$$

		TABLE 4-1	
		Multiplying by 10, 100, or 1000	
MULTIPLIER	NUMBER OF ZEROS	MOVE THE DECIMAL TO THE RIGHT	
10	1	1 place	
100	2	2 places	
1000	3	3 places	

✛ DIVISION OF DECIMALS

Division of Decimal Numbers

Division of decimals is done using the same method as is used for division of whole numbers. The special concern is movement and placement of the decimal point in the divisor (number divided by), dividend (number divided), and quotient (product).

$$\text{Divisor }\overline{)\text{Dividend}}^{\text{Quotient}} \qquad \frac{\text{Dividend}}{\text{Divisor}} = \text{Quotient}$$

$$8\overline{)64}^{\,8} \qquad \frac{64}{8} = 8$$

There will be few instances where you will be dividing decimals to calculate dosage problems. When you have to divide decimals, the most important thing to remember is placement of the decimal in the quotient. Review this helpful rule.

> ▶ RULE: To divide a decimal by a whole number, place the decimal point in the quotient directly above the decimal point in the dividend.

EXAMPLE: $25.5 \div 5$

$$\begin{array}{r} 5.1 \\ 5\overline{)25.5} \\ \underline{25} \\ 5 \\ \underline{5} \end{array}$$

Answer = 5.1

> ➤ RULE: To divide a decimal by a decimal,
> follow these steps:

- Make the decimal number in the divisor a
  whole number *first*. If you want to divide
  0.32 by 1.6, you would make 1.6 a whole
  number (16) by moving the decimal point 1
  place to the right.
- Move the decimal point in the dividend
  (0.32) the same number of places (1) that you
  moved the decimal point in the divisor.
- Place the decimal point in the quotient
  directly above the decimal point in the
  dividend.
- Divide 3.2 by 16.

$$16\overline{)3.2}^{\,.2}$$
$$3.2$$

Answer = 0.2

✛ DIVISION BY 10, 100, OR 1000

Dividing by 10, 100, or 1000 is fast and easy. Just
move the decimal point the same number of places
to the left as there are zeros in the divisor. See
Table 4-2.

EXAMPLE: 0.09 ÷ 10. Move the decimal one
place to the left for an answer of
0.009.

0.09 = .009 = 0.009

TABLE 4-2 Dividing by 10, 100, or 1000		
DIVISOR	NUMBER OF ZEROS	MOVE THE DECIMAL TO THE LEFT
10	1	1 place
100	2	2 places
1000	3	3 places

➤ *PRACTICE PROBLEMS* ➤

Add the following decimals:

1. $16.4 + 21.8 =$ _____

2. $0.009 + 18.4 =$ _____

3. $67.541 + 17.1 =$ _____

Subtract the following decimals:

4. $366.18 - 122.6 =$ _____

5. $107.16 - 56.1 =$ _____

6. $16.19 - 3.86 =$ _____

Multiply the following decimals:

7. $1.86 \times 12.1 =$ _____

8. $0.89 \times 7.65 =$ _____

9. $13 \times 7.8 =$ _____

10. $10.65 \times 100 =$ _____

Divide the following decimals:

11. $63.8 \div 0.09 =$_____

12. $39.7 \div 1.3 =$_____

13. $98.4 \div 1000 =$ _____

14. $0.008 \div 10 =$ _____

⊕ CHANGING FRACTIONS TO DECIMALS

Some fractions may divide evenly when converted into decimals. For example, the fraction 1/4 converts into 0.25, and 1/2 converts into 0.50. If a numerator does not divide evenly into the denominator, then work the division to three places.

$$\frac{1}{6} = \frac{\text{numerator}}{\text{denominator}} \quad \begin{matrix}\text{becomes}\\ \text{becomes}\end{matrix} \quad \frac{\text{dividend}}{\text{divisor}} = \frac{1}{6} \quad 6\overline{)1}$$

> ► RULE: To convert a fraction to a decimal, divide the numerator by the denominator. Follow these steps:

- Rewrite the fraction in the division format as shown previously; reduce if necessary.

$$6\overline{)1}$$

- Place a decimal point after the whole number in the dividend.
- Add zeros as needed.

$$6\overline{)1.0}$$

- Place the decimal point in the quotient directly above the decimal point in the dividend.

$$6\overline{)1.0}$$

- Divide.

EXAMPLES:

$$\frac{1}{8} = 1 \div 8 = 8\overline{)1}$$

$$\begin{array}{r} .125 \\ 8\overline{)1.000} \\ \underline{8} \\ 20 \\ \underline{16} \\ 40 \\ \underline{40} \end{array}$$

Answer = 0.125

$$\frac{5}{20} = \frac{1}{4} = 1 \div 4 = 4\overline{)1}$$

$$\begin{array}{r} .25 \\ 4\overline{)1.00} \\ \underline{8} \\ 20 \\ \underline{20} \end{array}$$

Answer = 0.25

$$\frac{6}{30} = \frac{1}{5} = 1 \div 5 = 5\overline{)1} \qquad 5\overline{)1.0} \\ \underline{10}$$

Answer = 0.2

⊕ CHANGING DECIMALS TO FRACTIONS

When changing decimals to fractions, the decimal number is expressed as a whole number and becomes the numerator of the fraction.

For example, $0.75 = \dfrac{75}{?}$. The denominator is expressed as the number 1 followed by zeros equal to the number of places to the right of the decimal fraction. For example:

1 place = a denominator of 10

2 places = a denominator of 100

3 places = a denominator of 1000

Therefore, 0.75 is expressed as 75/100.

> ► RULE: To change a decimal to a fraction, follow these steps:

- The decimal number becomes the numerator expressed as a whole number.
- The denominator is expressed as the number 1.

- The number of places to the right of the decimal point determines the number of zeros in the denominator.
- The common fraction is written and reduced if necessary.

EXAMPLE: 0.5   The number 5 becomes the numerator.

$$\frac{5}{?}$$

There is one place to the right of the decimal, which equals a denominator of 10.

The fraction becomes $\frac{5}{10} = \frac{1}{2}$

⊕ ROUNDING OFF DECIMALS

Most decimals are "rounded off" to the hundredth place to ensure accuracy of calculations. Because this process is done infrequently in the clinical setting, it is explained in Appendix A for those of you who wish to review the steps.

➤ *PRACTICE PROBLEMS* ➤

Convert the following fractions to decimals:

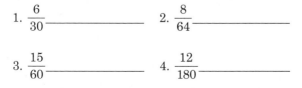

1. $\frac{6}{30}$ _____   2. $\frac{8}{64}$ _____

3. $\frac{15}{60}$ _____   4. $\frac{12}{180}$ _____

5. $\dfrac{16}{240}$ —————————

Convert the following decimals to fractions:

6. 0.007 _____   7. 0.93 _____

8. 0.412 _____   9. 5.03 _____

10. 12.2 _____

END OF CHAPTER REVIEW

Write the following decimals as you would read them:

1. 5.04 _____   2. 10.65 _____

3. 0.008 _____

Write the following decimals:

4. Six and eight hundredths

_____

5. One hundred twenty-four and three tenths

_____

6. Sixteen and one thousandths

_____

Solve the following decimal problems:

7. $16.35 + 8.1 =$ _____

8. $0.062 + 59.2 =$ _____

9. $7.006 - 4.23 =$ _____

10. $15.610 - 10.4 =$ _____

11. $27.05 \times 8.3 =$ _____

12. $0.009 \times 14.2 =$ _____

13. $18.75 \div 12 =$ _____

14. $1.070 \div 0.20 =$ _____

Convert the following fractions to decimals and decimals to fractions:

15. $\dfrac{6}{10}$ _____   16. $\dfrac{8}{20}$ _____

17. $\dfrac{12}{84}$ _____   18. $\dfrac{2}{9}$ _____

19. $\dfrac{3}{4}$ _____   20. $\dfrac{4}{5}$ _____

21. 0.45 _____   22. 6.8 _____

23. 0.75 _____   24. 1.35 _____

25. 0.06 _____   26. 8.5 _____

5

Percent, Ratio, and Proportion

The use of percentages is common to many disciplines and frequently encountered in the medical and nursing professions. Physicians prescribe solutions for external application (soaks, compresses) as well as internal use (gargling, irrigations, intravenous infusions). Nurses find themselves, sometimes daily, working with drugs and solutions prepared in percentage strength.

Today, pharmacists prepare most percentage-strength solutions; in fact, many that are used for external application are prepackaged by pharmaceutical companies. However, some institutions and home health care settings still require the preparation of solutions by nurses, and this will be covered in Chapter 16. This chapter will focus on the basic mathematical skills necessary to calculate percentage problems and will provide the foundation for understanding the preparation of solutions.

PERCENTS

A *percent*

- Refers to the number of units of something compared to the whole.

- Is always a division of 100.
- Means the "hundredth part."
- Is written with the symbol %, which means 100.
- When written as a solution, the % means "grams *per* 100 mL." A 5% solution means 5 grams of drug per 100 mL.
- Can be written as:
  - A fraction with a denominator of 100.
  - A decimal, by taking the unit to the hundredth part.

The *percent symbol* can be found with:

- A whole number   20%
- A fraction number   1/2%
- A mixed number   20 1/2%
- A decimal number   20.5%

✥ FRACTIONS AND PERCENTS

Sometimes it will be necessary to change a percent to a fraction or a fraction to a percent to make dosage calculations easier.

Changing a Percent to a Fraction

> ▶ RULE: To change a percent to a fraction, follow these steps:

- Drop the % symbol. 20% → 20
- Divide the number by 100. 20 ÷ 100 = 1/5

- Reduce the fraction to its lowest terms.
- Change it to a mixed number if necessary.

EXAMPLE: 40%

Change: $40\% = 40 = \dfrac{40}{100}$

Reduce: $\dfrac{40}{100} = \dfrac{2}{5}$

$$Answer = \dfrac{2}{5}$$

EXAMPLE: $\dfrac{1}{2}\%$

Change: $\dfrac{1}{2}\% = \dfrac{1}{2} = \dfrac{1/2}{100}$

$$\dfrac{1}{2} \div 100 = \dfrac{1}{2} \times \dfrac{1}{100} = \dfrac{1}{200}$$

$$Answer = \dfrac{1}{200}$$

Changing a Fraction to a Percent

> ► RULE: To change a fraction to a percent, follow these steps:

- Multiply the fraction by 100. For 1/2, multiply $1/2 \times 100 = 100/2$.
- Reduce if necessary. 100/2 = 50
- Add % symbol. 50%
- Change any improper fraction to a mixed number before multiplying by 100.

EXAMPLE: $\dfrac{3}{4}$

Change: $\dfrac{3}{4_1} \times \overset{25}{\cancel{100}} = \dfrac{75}{1} = 75$

Add % symbol: 75%

Answer = 75%

EXAMPLE: $\dfrac{3}{5}$

Change: $\dfrac{3}{5} \times 100 = \dfrac{3}{\cancel{5}_1} \times \overset{20}{\cancel{100}}_1 = 60$

Add % symbol: 60%

Answer = 60%

EXAMPLE: $6\dfrac{1}{2}$

Change: $6\dfrac{1}{2} \times 100$

Change $6\dfrac{1}{2}$ to an improper fraction.

$6\dfrac{1}{2} = \dfrac{13}{2}$

$\dfrac{13}{2} \times 100 = \dfrac{13}{\cancel{2}_1} \times \overset{50}{\cancel{100}}_1 = 650$

Add % symbol: 650%

Answer = 650%

➤ *PRACTICE PROBLEMS* ➤

Change the following percents to fractions:

1. 15%_____   2. 30%_____

3. 50%_____   4. 75%_____

5. 25%_____   6. 60%_____

Change the following fractions to percents:

7. $\dfrac{1}{3}$ _____   8. $\dfrac{2}{3}$ _____

9. $\dfrac{1}{5}$ _____   10. $\dfrac{3}{4}$ _____

11. $\dfrac{2}{5}$ _____   12. $\dfrac{1}{4}$ _____

⊕ DECIMALS AND PERCENTS

Sometimes it will be necessary to change a percent to a decimal or a decimal to a percent to make dosage calculations easier.

Changing a Percent to a Decimal

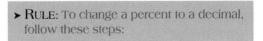

> ➤ RULE: To change a percent to a decimal, follow these steps:

♦ Drop the % symbol. When you drop a % symbol from a whole number, a decimal point takes the place of the symbol. For example, when you drop the % symbol from 68%, the decimal point replaces the % symbol (68.0).

- Divide by 100 by moving the decimal point two places to the left.

$$68.0 = .68. = 0.68$$

- Add zeros as needed.

EXAMPLE: 36%

Change: 36% = 36̶%̶ = 36.   decimal replaces % symbol

36. = .36. = 0.36   move the decimal point to the left

Answer = 0.36

EXAMPLE: 14.1%

14.1% = 14.1̶%̶ = 14.1

14.1 = .14.1 = 0.141

Answer = 0.141

Changing a Decimal to a Percent

> ► RULE: To change a decimal to a percent, follow these steps:

* Multiply by 100 by moving the decimal point two places to the right. For 3.19 you would move the decimal point two places to the right.

$$3.19 = 3.19. = 319$$
$$\llcorner\uparrow$$

* Add the % symbol: 319 = 319%
* Add zeros if needed.

EXAMPLE: 1.61

$1.61 \times 100 = 1.61. = 161$
$$\llcorner\uparrow$$

161 = 161%

Answer = 161%

EXAMPLE: 0.032

$0.032 \times 100 = 0.03.2 = 3.2$
$$\llcorner\uparrow$$

3.2 = 3.2%

Answer = 3.2%

➤ PRACTICE PROBLEMS ➤

Change the following percents to decimals:

1. 15%_____   2. 25%_____

3. 59%_____   4. 80%_____

Change the following decimals to percents:

5. 0.25_____   6. 0.45_____

7. 0.60_____   8. 0.85_____

⟐ RATIO AND PROPORTION

A ratio is used to express a relationship between two units or quantities. A slash (/) or colon (:) is used to indicate division, and both are read as "is to" or "per." A ratio is the same as a fraction! With medications, a ratio usually refers to the weight of a drug (eg, grams) in a solution (eg, mLs). Therefore, 50 mg/mL = 50 mg of a drug (solute) in 1 mL of a liquid (solution).

For the ratio of 1 is to 2, you can write 1:2 or 1/2. The *numerator (N) of the fraction is always to the left* of the colon or slash, and the *denominator (D) of the fraction is always to the right* of the colon or slash.

EXAMPLES: $N : D = N/D = \dfrac{N}{D}$

$$1 : 2 = 1/2 = \frac{1}{2}$$

A *proportion* states that two ratios are equal. A proportion can be written one of two ways. In the fraction form, the numerator and the denominator of one fraction have the same relationship as the numerator and denominator of another fraction. The equal symbol (=) is read as "as."

EXAMPLE: $\left.\dfrac{1}{3} = \dfrac{3}{9}\right\}$ 1 is to 3 as 3 is to 9

In the colon form, the ratio to the left of the double colon is equal to the ratio to the right of the double colon. The double colon (::) is read as "as."

EXAMPLE: 1:3 :: 3:9}   1 is to 3 as 3 is to 9

With the example, the first and fourth terms are called *extremes,* while the second and third terms are called the *means.*

EXTREMES

$$\overbrace{1{:}3 :: 3{:}9}$$

MEANS

> ► RULE: In a proportion, the product of the means is always equal to the product of the extremes.

To verify that two ratios in a proportion are equal:

- *For a fraction,* multiply the numerator of each ratio by its opposite denominator. The sum products will be equal.

EXAMPLE: $\dfrac{1}{3} : \dfrac{3}{9}$

$$\dfrac{1}{3} : \dfrac{3}{9}$$

$$1 \times 9 = 9$$

$$3 \times 3 = 9$$

$$9 = 9$$

- *For a ratio,* multiply the means and then multiply the extremes.

The product of the means equals the product of the extremes.

EXAMPLE: 1:3 :: 3:9

$$\overbrace{1:3 :: 3:9}$$

$$1 \times 9 = 9$$

$$3 \times 3 = 9$$

$$9 = 9$$

⊕ USE OF RATIO AND PROPORTION: SOLVING FOR *X*

In review, a *ratio* expresses the relationship of one unit/quantity to another. A *proportion* expresses the relationship between two ratios that are equal. When a proportion has one unknown quantity, known as *x,* you can calculate for that quantity by using ratio and proportion and *solving for x.*

USE OF RATIOS AND PROPORTIONS: SOLVING FOR *X*

Using the previous examples of 1/3 = 3/9, assume that one number is unknown.

EXAMPLE: $\dfrac{1}{3} = \dfrac{x}{9}$ x = unknown

> ► **RULE:** Cross-multiply the denominator on the left with the numerator on the right. Cross-multiply the denominator on the right with the numerator on the left. Divide both sides of the equation by the number before the *x.*

Cross-multiply: $3 \times x = 9 \times 1$

                         $3x = 9$

Divide both sides of the equation by the number before the *x.*

$$3x = 9$$

Divide: $$\frac{\overset{1}{\cancel{3}}x}{\cancel{3}_1} = \frac{\cancel{9}^3}{\cancel{3}_1}$$

Reduce: $$x = \frac{3}{1}$$

$$x = 3$$

Note: Because the number *before* the x is the same in the numerator and denominator of one ratio, these numbers will cross themselves out and equal 1. Therefore, a shortcut is to *move the number before the x to the denominator on the opposite side.* This quick process is especially important when solving for x in dosage calculation problems.

In order to understand how to apply the concept of *solving for x,* using ratios and proportions, for drug dosage problems presented in Chapters 11 and 12, a medication example will be presented here.

USE OF RATIO AND PROPORTION: SOLVING FOR X USING A MEDICATION EXAMPLE

Frequently in dosage calculation problems, one quantity is known (eg, 100 mg per mL = 100 mg/1 mL), and it is necessary to find an unknown quantity because the physician has ordered something different from what is available (eg, 75 mg). In a proportion problem, the unknown quantity (? mL to give for 75 mg) is identified as x.

Read the following word problem and solve for x.

EXAMPLE: Demerol in 75 milligrams is prescribed for postoperative pain. The medication is available as 100 milligrams in 1 milliliter. To administer the prescribed dose of 75 milligrams, the nurse would give _____ milliliter(s).

> ► RULE: To solve for x using a fraction format, follow the steps below:

♦ Write down what is available or *what you have* in a fraction format. You are expressing the relationship of one quantity (mg) to another quantity (mL). *Remember,* the unit of measurement in the numerator of the fraction must be the same for both fractions. The unit of measurement in the denominator of the fraction also must be the same for both fractions.

EXAMPLE: You should write:

$$\frac{100 \text{ mg}}{1 \text{ mL}}$$

♦ Complete the proportion by writing down what you desire in a fraction format, making sure that the numerators are like units and the denominators are like units:

$$\frac{\text{mg}}{\text{mL}} :: \frac{\text{mg}}{\text{mL}} = \frac{100 \text{ mg}}{1 \text{ mL}} :: \frac{75 \text{ mg}}{x \text{ mL}}$$

- *Cross-multiply* the numerator of each fraction by its opposite denominator and drop the terms used for units of measurement.

$$\frac{100 \text{ mg}}{1 \text{ mL}} \diagdown \underset{\cdot\cdot}{\diagup} \frac{75 \text{ mg}}{x \text{ mL}}$$

By doing this, you should get the following proportion:

$$100 \times x = 75 \times 1$$

$$100x = 75$$

- Solve for x by dividing both sides of the equation by the number before x. In this case, the number before x is 100, so divide both sides of the equation by 100. Convert your answer to a decimal, which is easier to work with than a fraction. Refer to pages 71–77 to review the traditional and abbreviated methods for solving for x. For the purpose of brevity, an abbreviated method will be used throughout the remainder of the book.

$$\frac{100x}{100} = \frac{75}{100}$$

$$x = \frac{75}{100}$$

Reduce: $\quad x = \dfrac{3}{4}$ mL or 0.75 mL

> ► RULE: To solve for x using a colon format, follow these steps:

EXAMPLE: Demerol in 75 milligrams is prescribed for postoperative pain. The
medication is available as 100 milligrams in 1 milliliter. To administer
the prescribed dose of 75 milligrams,
the nurse would have to give
_____ milliliter(s).

- Write down what is available or *what you
  have* in colon format. *Remember,* the unit of
  measurement to the left of the colon must be
  the same for both ratios; the unit of
  measurement to the right of the colon must
  be the same for both ratios. For this
  example, you should write:

  100 mg : 1 mL

- Complete the proportion by writing down
  what you desire, in a colon format, making
  sure that both ratios are written in the same
  format.

  100 mg : 1 mL :: 75 mg : x mL

- Multiply the extremes:

  ┌─────EXTREMES─────┐
  100 mg : 1 mL :: 75 mg : x mL

  (100 mg × x mL =   )

- Multiply the means:

$$100 \text{ mg} : 1 \text{ mL} :: 75 \text{ mg} : x \text{ mL}$$

$$\underline{\quad\text{MEANS}\quad}$$

($\quad$ = 75 mg × 1 mL)

- Complete the equation 100 mg × x mL = 75 mg × 1 mL and drop the units of measurement.

$$100x = 75$$

- Solve for x. (Remember, divide both sides of the equation by the number before x [100].) Convert your answer to a decimal.

$$\frac{100x}{100} = \frac{75}{100}$$

$$\frac{\cancel{100}x}{\cancel{100}} = \frac{75}{100}$$

Reduce: $\quad x = \dfrac{3}{4} \text{ mL or } 0.75 \text{ mL}$

Answer = 0.75 mL

- Verify the accuracy of the answer, $x = 0.75$ mL.
- For the fraction format, multiply the numerator of each ratio by its opposite denominator. The sum products will be equal.

$$\frac{100 \text{ mg}}{1 \text{ mL}} :: \frac{75 \text{ mg}}{\frac{3}{4} \text{ mL}}$$

$$\overset{25}{\cancel{100}} \times \frac{3}{4_1} = 75$$

$$1 \times 75 = 75$$

} Sum products are equal

- For the colon format, multiply the means and then multiply the extremes. The product of the means will equal the product of the extremes.

┌─────EXTREMES─────┐

100 mg : 1 mL :: 75 mg : $\frac{3}{4}$ mL

└─MEANS─┘

$$75 \times 1 = 75$$

$$100 \times \frac{3}{4} = \frac{\overset{25}{\cancel{100}}}{1} \times \frac{3}{4_1} = 75$$

} Sum products are equal

➤ PRACTICE PROBLEMS ➤

Write the following relationships in ratio form, using both the fraction and colon format:

1. Amoxil pediatric drops contain 50 milligrams of amoxicillin in 5 milliliters of solution.
2. There are 325 milligrams of acetaminophen in 1 tablet of Tylenol.
3. Each liter of dextrose solution contains 2 ampules of multivitamins.

Write the following relationships as proportions, using both the fraction and colon format:

4. Each aspirin tablet contains 5 grains of acetyl-salicylic acid (ASA). The nurse is to give 3 aspirin tablets equal to 15 grains of ASA.
5. Catapres is available in 0.2 milligram tablets. A patient was prescribed 0.4 milligrams/day provided by 2 tablets.
6. Alupent is available in syrup form as 10 milligrams/5 milliliters. A patient is to take 30 milligrams or 15 milliliters during a 24-hour period.

Use ratios and proportions to solve for x.

7. $\dfrac{4}{12} = \dfrac{3}{x}$ _____   8. $\dfrac{6}{x} = \dfrac{9}{27}$ _____

9. $\dfrac{2}{7} = \dfrac{x}{14}$ _____

10. If 50 mg of a drug is available in 1 mL of solution, how many milliliters would contain 40 mg?

Set up ratio: proportion with x:_____

Solve for x: _____

11. Promethazine hydrochloride is available as 25 mg/mL.

To give 1.5 mL, you would give _____ mg.

Set up ratio: proportion with x:_____

Solve for x: _____

12. Lanoxin in 0.125 mg is available per tablet.

The nurse gave 2 tablets or _____ mg.

Set up ratio: proportion with x:_____

Solve for x: _____

END OF CHAPTER REVIEW

Change the following:

	Percent	Fraction	Decimal
1.	_____	1/6	_____
2.	_____		0.25
3.	6.4%	_____	_____
4.	21%	_____	_____

5. _____	2/5	_____
6. _____	_____	1.62
7. _____	_____	0.27
8. 5 1/4%	_____	_____
9. _____	9/2	_____
10. 8 3/9%	_____	_____
11. 1%	_____	_____
12. _____	6/7	_____
13. _____	18/4	_____
14. _____	_____	1.5
15. _____	_____	0.72

Write the following ratios in fraction and colon format:

16. Chewable Cardilate tablets contain 10 milligrams of erythrityl tetranitrate in each tablet.

_____ fraction   _____ colon

17. Pitocin is available for injection as 10 units in each milliliter.

_____ fraction   _____ colon

18. For a serious infection, a physician could prescribe 200 milligrams of azlocillin for every kilogram of body weight.

_____ fraction   _____ colon

19. The physician ordered 300 milligrams of quinidine sulfate. The tablets were available in 100 milligrams per tablet.

_____ fraction   _____ colon

20. Dymelor in 500 milligrams was ordered for a patient every morning. The medication was available in 250-milligram tablets.

_____ fraction   _____ colon

21. Synthroid is available in 0.075-milligram tablets. A physician ordered 0.15 milligrams daily.

_____ fraction   _____ colon

Solve for x, using ratios and proportions.

22. If $\dfrac{1}{50} = \dfrac{x}{40}$ then $x =$

23. If $\dfrac{6}{18} = \dfrac{2}{x}$ then $x =$

24. If $\dfrac{x}{12} = \dfrac{9}{24}$ then $x =$

25. If $\dfrac{3}{9} = \dfrac{x}{18}$ then $x =$

Solve for x for the remaining problems and verify your answers using a fraction or colon format:

26. The physician prescribed 10 milligrams of Vasoxyl for moderate postoperative hypotension. The medication was available as 20 milligrams in 1 milliliter. The nurse would give _____ milliliter(s).

Verify your answer: _____

27. The physician prescribed 25 milligrams of meperidine hydrochloride syrup to be given every 3 hours for pain as needed. The syrup preparation was available as 50 milligrams in 5 milliliters. To give 25 milligrams, the nurse would give _____ milliliter(s).

Verify your answer: _____

28. The physician ordered 1.5 milligrams of leucovorin calcium for nutritional deficiency. The medication was available as 3.0 milligrams in a 1.0-milliliter ampule. The nurse would give _____ milliliter(s).

Verify your answer: _____

29. The physician prescribed 35 milligrams of furosemide (Lasix) as a one-dose, intramuscular injection for diuresis. The medication was available as 20 milligrams in 2 milliliters. The nurse would give _____ milliliter(s).

Verify your answer: _____

30. The physician prescribed 30 milligrams of fluoxetine hydrochloride (Prozac) to be given _____ for depression. The oral solution was available as 20 milligrams in 5 milliliters. The nurse would give _____ milliliter(s).

31. The physician prescribed 40 milligrams of Elixophyllin solution for relief of bronchial asthma. The medication was available as 80 milligrams in 15 milliliters. To give 40 milligrams, the nurse would give _____ milliliters.

32. The physician prescribed 7.5 milligrams of morphine for severe pain. The medication was available as 15 milligrams in 1 milliliter. The nurse would give _____ milliliters.

33. The physician prescribed 0.6 milligrams of atropine sulfate, preoperatively. The medication was available as 0.4 milligrams in 1 milliliter. To give 0.6 milligrams, the nurse would give _____ milliliter(s).

34. The physician prescribed 80 milligrams of Dilantin by injection to treat psychomotor seizures. The medication was available as 100 milligrams in 2 milliliters. The nurse would give _____ milliliter(s).

End of Unit I Review

Solve the following problems and reduce each answer to its lowest terms.

1. 1/4 + 3/4 _____

2. 2/3 − 3/5 _____

3. 1/10 + 3/5 _____

4. 3/4 − 1/3 _____

5. 2/6 × 4/5 _____

6. 3/8 × 1/6 _____

7. 1/50 × 20/30 _____

8. 1/100 × 20/30 _____

9. 1/3 ÷ 1/6 _____

10. 1/10 ÷ 1/8 _____

11. 1/12 ÷ 1/3 _____

12. 1/15 ÷ 3/150 _____

Choose the fraction with the highest value in each of the following.

13. 1/3 or 1/4 _____

14. 1/8 or 1/6 _____

15. 1/100 or 1/200 _____

16. 3/30 or 5/30 _____

Solve the following and carry to the nearest hundredths.

17. 1.5 + 1.6 _____

18. 0.46 + 3.8 _____

19. 0.6 − 0.2 _____

20. 6 − 0.32 _____

21. 0.25 × 10 _____

22. 0.15 × 100 _____

23. 7.5 ÷ 0.45 _____

24. 8.5 ÷ 4.5 _____

Change the following fractions to decimals and decimals to fractions.

25. 8/10 _____   26. 5/20 _____

27. 3/9 _____   28. 0.5 _____

29. 0.07 _____   30. 1.5 _____

Change the following percents to fractions and fractions to percents.

31. 25% _____   32. 1/3% _____

33. 0.6% _____   34. 2/5 _____

35. 4 1/2 _____   36. 1/50 _____

Solve for the value of x in each ratio and proportion problem. Reduce all fractions to their lowest terms or carry all decimals to the hundredths.

37. $3 : x :: 4 : 16$ _____

38. $25 : 1.5 :: 20 : x$ _____

39. $8 : 1 :: 10 : x$ _____

40. $4/5 : 25 :: x : 50$ _____

41. $0.25 : 500 :: x : 1000$ _____

42. $x : 20 :: 2.5 : 100$ _____

Measurement Systems

The metric and apothecaries' systems of weights and measures are in wide use today, as they have been for many years. While the apothecaries' system is still used today by many health care practitioners, with the current shift in health delivery from the institution to the home, the use of household measurements also is becoming more popular.

To effectively deliver medications today, nurses need to be familiar with all three systems of measurement and to become expert at converting one unit of measure to another, within the same system, or between two systems. This unit will present the metric and apothecaries' systems as well as the household measurements. The reader will be shown how to convert all measurements. Equivalent values have been listed to facilitate conversions and dosage calculations.

6

The Metric System/International System of Units/SI

The metric system, a decimal system based on weights and measures, is based on the *meter* (approximately equal to a yard). All units differ in multiples of ten. Portions can be increased or decreased by multiples of ten (10, 100, 1000). Conversions are achieved by moving the decimal point to the right for multiplication or to the left for division.

$$1.0 \ \textit{increased by} \ 10 = 1.0. = 10$$

$$0.1 \ \textit{decreased by} \ 10 = 0.1 = 0.01$$

The metric system has three basic units of measurement: length (meter), volume (liter), and weight (gram). Three common prefixes are used to indicate units of measure:

micro = one millionth = mc
milli = one thousandth = m
centi = one hundredth = c

One prefix, used to indicate a larger unit of measurement, is frequently used to measure body weight:

$$\text{kilo} = \text{one thousand} = \text{k}$$

⊕ COMMON RULES FOR METRIC NOTATIONS

- Metric abbreviations always follow Arabic numerals.

    0.2 mL   10 kg

- Basic units are written in lowercase letters except for the word *liter;* the "L" is capitalized.

    g = gram

    mL = milliliter

- Fractional units are expressed as decimal fractions.

    0.5 mL *not* 1/2 mL

- Zeros are only used *in front of* the decimal point, when not preceded by a whole number, to emphasize the decimal. (Omit unnecessary zeros so the dosage is not misread).

    0.5 mL *not* 0.50 mL

    1 mL *not* 1.0 mL

⊕ METER—LENGTH

A meter is:

* The basic unit of length
* Equal to 39.37 inches
* Abbreviated as m

The primary linear measurements used in medicine are centimeters and millimeters. Centimeters are used for measuring such things as the size of body organs and wounds; millimeters are used for blood pressure measurements. The important units of metric length are found in Table 6-1.

You can move about from point to point in the metric system.

> ► RULE: To move from smaller to larger units, follow these steps:

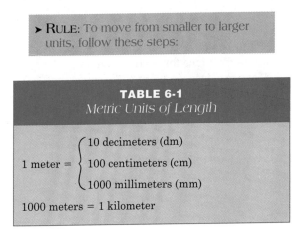

TABLE 6-1
Metric Units of Length

$$1 \text{ meter} = \begin{cases} 10 \text{ decimeters (dm)} \\ 100 \text{ centimeters (cm)} \\ 1000 \text{ millimeters (mm)} \end{cases}$$

1000 meters = 1 kilometer

- Count the number of places to be moved.
  Move one place for each increment of 10.
- Move the decimal point to the left the
  number of places counted.

EXAMPLE: Change millimeters (6000) to decime-
             ters. To move from milli to deci, you
             need to move two places to the left.

             60.00. = 60

             (milli) = (deci)

                                    Answer = 60 dm

> ► RULE: To move from larger to smaller
>   units, follow these steps:

- Count the number of places to be moved.
  Move one place for each increment of 10.
- Move the decimal point *to the right* the
  number of places counted.

EXAMPLE: Change deci (80) to centi. To move
             from deci to centi, you need to move
             one place. Count one place to the
             right.

             80.0. = 800

             (deci) = (centi)

                                    Answer = 800 cm

➤ PRACTICE PROBLEMS ➤

Change the following units of metric length:

1. 3.60 cm = _____ m

2. 4.16 m = _____ dm

3. 0.8 mm = _____ cm

4. 2 mm = _____ m

⊕ LITER—VOLUME

A liter is:

- The basic unit of volume
- The total volume of liquid in a cube that measures 10 cm × 10 cm × 10 cm (= cm³) (see Figure 6-1)
- Equal to 1000 mL = 1000 cc
- Abbreviated as L

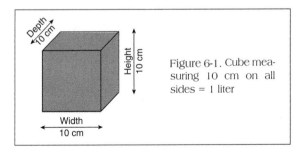

Figure 6-1. Cube measuring 10 cm on all sides = 1 liter

It is important to note that 1 liter equals 1000 mL, which also equals 1000 cc. A cc is the amount of space occupied by 1 mL of volume. The units of metric volume can be found in Table 6-2.

The rules for moving from larger to smaller and from smaller to larger units of metric length can also be used for units of metric volume and weight.

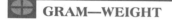 GRAM—WEIGHT

A gram is:

+ The basic unit of weight.
+ The weight of distilled water in 1 cubic centimeter at a temperature of 4°C.
+ A cube 1 cm^3 (see Figure 6-2).
+ Equal to a volume of 1 mL in cc.
+ Abbreviated as g.

The units of metric weight can be found in Table 6-3.

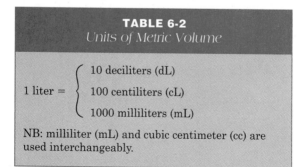

TABLE 6-2
Units of Metric Volume

$$1 \text{ liter} = \begin{cases} 10 \text{ deciliters (dL)} \\ 100 \text{ centiliters (cL)} \\ 1000 \text{ milliliters (mL)} \end{cases}$$

NB: milliliter (mL) and cubic centimeter (cc) are used interchangeably.

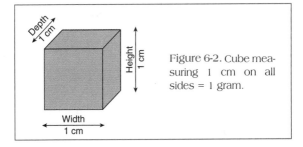

Figure 6-2. Cube measuring 1 cm on all sides = 1 gram.

➤ PRACTICE PROBLEMS ➤

Change the following units of metric volume and weight:

1. 3.006 mL = _____ L

2. 6.17 cL = _____ mL

3. 0.9 L = _____ mL

4. 6.40 cg = _____ mg

5. 1000 mg = _____ g

6. 0.8 mg = _____ dg

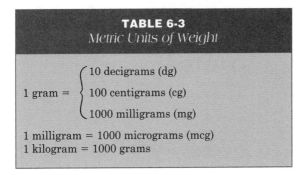

TABLE 6-3
Metric Units of Weight

$$1 \text{ gram} = \begin{cases} 10 \text{ decigrams (dg)} \\ 100 \text{ centigrams (cg)} \\ 1000 \text{ milligrams (mg)} \end{cases}$$

1 milligram = 1000 micrograms (mcg)
1 kilogram = 1000 grams

END OF CHAPTER REVIEW

Change the following units of metric length:

1. 7.43 mm = _____ m   2. 0.06 cm = _____ dm

3. 10 km = _____ m   4. 62.17 dm = ___ mm

Change the following units of metric volume:

5. 1.64 mL = _____ dL   6. 0.47 dL = _____ L

7. 10 L = _____ cL   8. 56.9 cL = _____ mL

Change the following units of metric weight:

9. 35.6 mg = _____ g   10. 0.3 g = _____ cg

11. 0.05 g = _____ mg   12. 93 cg = _____ mg

13. 100 mcg = _____ mg   14. 2 mg = _____ mcg

15. 1.0 mcg = _____ mg   16. 7 kg = _____ g

Perform the following miscellaneous conversions:

17. 4 mg = _____ mcg   18. 13 kg = _____ g

19. 2.5 L = _____ mL   20. 0.6 mg = _____ mcg

21. 0.08 g = _____ mg   22. 0.01 mg = _____ mcg

7

The Apothecaries' System

One of the oldest systems of measurement is the apothecaries' system. While less popular than the metric system, it is still used by physicians, especially for prescribing medications that have been used for many years (eg, digitalis, aspirin).

The apothecaries' system has two basic units of measurement (see Tables 7-1 and 7-2).

UNIT	TERM
Weight	Grain = gr
Volume	Minim = m
	Dram = ʒ or dr
	Ounce = ℥ or oz

A grain is equal to the weight of a grain of wheat; the minim is equal to the quantity of water in a drop that also weighs 1 grain. A dram is equal to 4 mL; an ounce is equal to 30 mL.

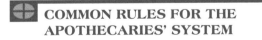 **COMMON RULES FOR THE APOTHECARIES' SYSTEM**

- Roman numerals are used to express numbers.
- The apothecaries' abbreviation *always goes before* the quantity.

TABLE 7-1
Apothecary Units of Weight

UNIT	WEIGHT	SYMBOL
Grain*	—	gr
Dram	60 grains	ʒ
Ounce	8 drams	℥ or oz
Pound	12 ounces†	lb

*The grain is the basic unit.
†A pound in this system is equal to 12 ounces; a pound in the English system is equal to 16 ounces.

TABLE 7-2
Apothecary Units of Volume

UNIT	VOLUME	SYMBOL
Minim*	1 drop of water	m or min
Fluidram†	60 minims	fʒ
Fluidounce†	8 fluidrams	f℥
Pint	16 fluidounces	pt or 0
Quart	2 pints	qt
Gallon	4 quarts	gal or C

*The minim is the basic unit.
†When the substance is known to be a liquid, the term fluid does not have to be used.

Examples: gr x̄ = grains 10
                  ʒ viii = eight drams

- Fractional units are used to express quantities that are less than one. They are written as common fractions, except for 1/2. The symbol ss or s̈s̈ is acceptable for 1/2.

EXAMPLES: gr $\dfrac{1}{2}$ or gr ss or gr s̈s̈

           gr $\dfrac{1}{300}$

- Roman or Arabic numerals can be used for large quantities or when the amount is to be written out.

EXAMPLES: ℨ xx or ℨ 20 = twenty drams

Sometimes it will be necessary to change from one unit to another within the same system.

> ► RULE: To change units within the same system, follow these steps:*

- Look up the equivalent values in the system. For example, if you want to know how many ounces there are in 20 drams, then look up the equivalent value of 8 drams = 1 ounce.
- Write down *what you know* in a ratio or fraction format:

EXAMPLE: $\dfrac{8 \text{ drams}}{1 \text{ ounce}}$

        or 8 drams : 1 ounce

---

*Refer to pages 71–77 to review solving for *x*.

- Write down *what you desire* in a ratio or fraction format to complete the proportion. The numerators and denominators must be the same units of measurement. The unknown value is referred to as x:

$$\frac{8 \text{ drams}}{1 \text{ ounce}} :: \frac{20 \text{ drams}}{x \text{ ounces}} \quad \text{or}$$

8 drams : x ounces :: 20 drams : 1 ounce

- Cross-multiply to get the following. Drop the terms used for units of measurement.

8 drams $\times$ x ounces = 20 drams $\times$ 1 ounce

$$8x = 20$$

- Solve for x (divide both sides of the equation by the number before the x [8]). You are reducing both sides of the equation.

$$\frac{8x}{8} = \frac{20}{8}$$

$$\frac{8^1 x}{8_1}$$

Reduce: $\quad x = \frac{20^5}{8_2}$

$$x = \frac{5}{2} = 2\frac{1}{2}$$

$$Answer = 2\frac{1}{2} \text{ ounces}$$

END OF CHAPTER REVIEW

Write the following, using Roman numerals and symbols:

1. 3 grains_____ 2. 5 drams _____

3. 8 fluidrams_____ 4. 10 minims _____

5. 20 1/2 minims_____ 6. 5 pints _____

Solve the following:

7. 8 quarts = _____ gallon(s)

8. f℥ ii = _____ minim(s)

9. f℥ iv = _____ fluidram(s)

10. gr xxx = _____ dram(s)

11. f℥ viii = _____ ounce(s)

12. 4 pints = _____ quart(s)

13. 4 ounces = _____ pint(s)

14. gr xv = _____ dram(s)

15. 1/4 ℥ = _____ dram(s)

16. ℥ ss̈ = _____ dram(s)

8

Household Measurements

Household measurements are calculated by using containers easily found in the home. Common household measuring devices are those utensils used for cooking, eating, and measuring liquid proportions. They include medicine droppers, teaspoons, tablespoons, cups, and glasses. Because containers differ in design, size, and capacity, it is impossible to establish a standard unit of measure. The household measurement system is the *least accurate* of all three systems, yet its use will increase as health care moves into the community. The nurse or health care worker may have to teach the patient/family how to measure the amount of medication prescribed, so every effort needs to be made to be as exact as possible.

Probably the *most common* measuring device found in the home is the measuring cup, which calibrates ounces and cups and is available for liquid and dry measures (Figure 8-1). Additionally, many families have a 1-ounce measuring cup that calibrates teaspoons and/or tablespoons (Figure 8-2). Some pharmaceutical companies package 1-ounce measuring cups or calibrated medicine droppers with their over-the-counter medications (NyQuil, Children's Tylenol).

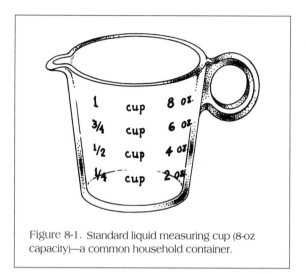

Figure 8-1. Standard liquid measuring cup (8-oz capacity)—a common household container.

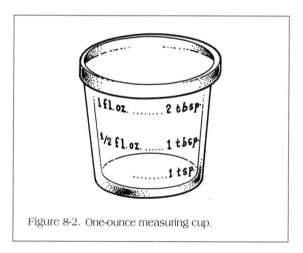

Figure 8-2. One-ounce measuring cup.

The household system of measurement uses Arabic whole numbers and fractions to express quantities. Standard cookbook abbreviations are used (tsp, tbsp, oz). Even though household measurements are approximate in comparison to the exactness of the metric and apothecaries' systems, they are frequently used and do have equivalent values in the other systems. Hospitals commonly used a standard 1-ounce measuring cup (Figure 8-3). The calibrated containers use the metric, apothecaries', and household systems and indicate the equivalent value in ounces.

The basic unit of this system is the drop (gtt). For consistency within the system, a drop is equal to a drop, regardless of the liquid's viscosity (sticky or gummy consistency).

When measuring a liquid medication, it is important that the container/dropper be held so the calibrations are at eye level. When a container/drop-

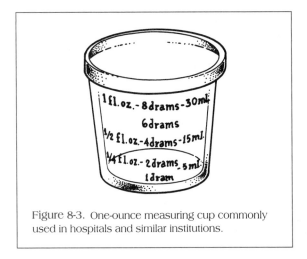

Figure 8-3. One-ounce measuring cup commonly used in hospitals and similar institutions.

per is held at eye level, the liquid will appear to be uneven or U-shaped. This curve, called a *meniscus,* is caused by surface tension; its shape is influenced by the viscosity of the fluid. When measuring the level of a liquid medication, read the calibration "at the bottom" of the meniscus (Figure 8-4).

> ➤ RULE: To change units within the same system, follow these steps:

+ Look up the equivalent values in the system (Table 8-1). If you want to know how many ounces there are in 4 tablespoons, then look up the equivalent value of 1 ounce = 2 tablespoons.

TABLE 8-1
Common Household Quantities

UNIT	VOLUME	SYMBOL
Drop	—	gtt
Teaspoon	60 drops	t or tsp
Tablespoon	3 teaspoons	T or tbs or tbsp
Ounce	2 tablespoons	oz
Cup	6 ounces*	c
Glass or cup	8 ounces	gl
Pint	16 ounces	pt
Quart	2 pints	qt

*Refers to a teacup, not a measuring cup.

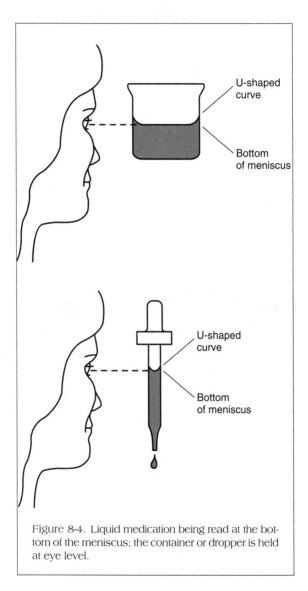

Figure 8-4. Liquid medication being read at the bottom of the meniscus; the container or dropper is held at eye level.

EXAMPLE: Write down *what you know* in a fraction or ratio format.

$$\left(\frac{2 \text{ tbs}}{1 \text{ oz}} \text{ or } 2 \text{ tbs} : 1 \text{ oz} \right)$$

◆ Write down *what you desire* in a fraction or ratio format to complete the proportion. The unknown unit is referred to as *x*. The numerator and denominator must be the same units of measurement. Consider the fraction format here.

$$\frac{2 \text{ tbs}}{1 \text{ oz}} : \frac{4 \text{ tbs}}{x \text{ oz}}$$

◆ Cross-multiply to get the following. Drop the terms used for units of measurement.

$$2 \text{ tbs} \times x \text{ oz} = 4 \text{ tbs} \times 1 \text{ oz}$$

$$2x = 4$$

Solve for x:

$$\frac{2x}{2} = \frac{4}{2}$$

$$\frac{\cancel{2}^1 x}{\cancel{2}_1} = \frac{\cancel{4}^2}{\cancel{2}_1}$$

$$x = 2$$

Answer = 2 ounces

END OF CHAPTER REVIEW

Convert the following units to their equivalent value:

1. 12 ounces = _____ cup(s)

2. 3 glasses = _____ ounces

3. 6 tablespoons = _____ ounce(s)

4. 2 teaspoons =_____ drops

5. 3 tablespoons = _____ teaspoons

6. 2 cups = _____ ounces

7. 8 ounces = _____ pint(s)

8. 2 glasses = _____ pint(s)

9. 2 ounces =_____ tablespoons

10. 1/4 cup =_____ ounces

11. 3/4 cup =_____ ounces

12. 3 pints = _____ quart(s)

13. 6 teaspoons = _____ ounce(s)

14. 2 pints = _____ ounces

15. 1/2 teaspoon = _____ drops

9

System Equivalents and System Conversions

Many times a drug is prescribed in a unit different from the unit that is available. Previous chapters (6, 7, and 8) have shown you how to change from one unit to another *within the same system*. This chapter will show you how to convert units from two different systems. To successfully convert between systems, you should memorize certain essential equivalent values among units. It must be remembered that equivalent values are just that, equivalent—almost but not quite equal. A common example of such a discrepancy is between the metric and apothecaries' systems. You will see that 60 mg or 65 mg = 1 grain. For example, a medication label will indicate 5 grains, and its equivalent dosage may be written as 300 mg or 325 mg. Both dosages are correct; the equivalent values are approximate.

To make conversions from one system to another easier, it is necessary to memorize the following equivalents (Table 9-1). When recording equivalent values, numerals are rounded off to facilitate drug calculations.

The metric and English household equivalents for length are rarely used for drug dosage calculations but can be used when applying a paste, cream, or ointment that needs to cover a certain area.

TABLE 9-1
Volume and Weight Equivalents

METRIC SYSTEM	APOTHECARIES' SYSTEM	HOUSEHOLD MEASUREMENTS
Volume		
—	1 minim	1 drop
1 milliliter	15–16 minims	15–16 drops
4–5 milliliters	1 dram (60 minims)	1 teaspoon (60 gtts)
15 milliliters	4 drams (3–4 teaspoons)	1 tablespoon (1/2 ounce)
30 milliliters	1 ounce (8 drams)	2 tablespoons (1 ounce)
180 milliliters	6 ounces	1 teacup
240 milliliters	8 ounces	1 glass/ measuring cup
500 milliliters	1 pint	1 pint (16 ounces)
1000 milliliters (1 liter)	1 quart	1 quart (32 ounces)
	2 pints	1 quart
	4 quarts	1 gallon
Weight		
0.60–0.65 milligrams	gr 1/100	—
0.5 milligrams	gr 1/120	—
0.4 milligrams	gr 1/150	—
0.3 milligrams	gr 1/200	—
0.2 milligrams	gr 1/300	—

TABLE 9-1 *(continued)*

METRIC SYSTEM	APOTHECARIES' SYSTEM	HOUSEHOLD MEASUREMENTS
Weight		
1000 micrograms	gr 1/60	—
1 mg (1000 mcg)	gr 1/60	—
4 mg	gr 1/15	—
6 mg	gr 1/10	—
10 mg	gr 1/6	—
15 mg	gr 1/4	—
60–65 milligrams	1 grain	—
1 gram (1000 mg)	15 grains	—
4–5 grams	1 dram	—
15 grams	4 drams	—
30 grams	8 drams	1 ounce
454 grams	12 ounces	1 pound
1 kilogram (1000 grams)		2.2 pounds

However, both are used for linear measurements, eg, to measure wound size, head circumference, abdominal girth, and height (Table 9-2).

TABLE 9-2
*Linear Equivalents for the Household
and Metric Systems*

HOUSEHOLD	METRIC
1 inch	2.5 centimeters
	25 millimeters
12 inches (1 foot)	30 centimeters
39.4 inches (1 yard + 3.4 inches)	1 meter

✛ SYSTEM CONVERSIONS USING VOLUME AND WEIGHT UNITS

> ▶ RULE: To solve for *x* when converting between systems, follow these steps:

♦ Look up the equivalent value between the systems. If you want to know how many grams there are in 30 grains, you would look up the equivalent value of 15 grains = 1 gram.

EXAMPLES:

♦ Write down *what you know* in a fraction or colon format.

15 grains : 1 gram

- Complete the proportion by writing down *what you desire.* Keep the units of measurement in the correct spaces.

15 grains : 1 gram :: 30 grains : x grams

$$15 \times x = 30 \times 1$$

- Multiply the extremes and then multiply the means. Drop the terms used for units of measurement.

$$15x = 30$$

- Solve for x:

$$\frac{15x}{15} = \frac{30}{15}$$

$$\frac{\cancel{15}^1 x}{\cancel{15}_1} = \frac{\cancel{30}^2}{\cancel{15}_1}$$

$$x = 2 \text{ grams}$$

Answer = 2 grams

➤ PRACTICE PROBLEMS ➤

Complete the following. Solve for x or the unknown by using a fraction or colon format.

1. 12 fluidrams = _____ milliliter(s)

2. 3 milliliters = _____ minim(s)

3. 2 teaspoons = _____ milliliter(s)

Complete the following. Solve for *x* or the unknown by using a fraction or colon format.

4. gr 1/200 = _____ milligram(s)

5. 6 drams = _____ gram(s)

6. 30 mL = _____ ounce(s)

7. 6 mg = _____ grain(s)

8. 1 liter = _____ quart(s)

9. 2.2 lb = _____ kilogram(s)

END OF CHAPTER REVIEW

Complete the following. Solve for *x* by using a fraction or colon format.

1. A child who weighs 55 pounds weighs _____ kilogram.
2. Two (2) ounces of Metamucil powder would be equivalent to _____ gram(s).
3. A patient is restricted to four 8-ounce glasses of water per day. The nurse knows that the patient's fluid intake is restricted to _____ milliliters per day.
4. A patient's abdominal wound measures 10 centimeters in diameter. The nurse knows this is equivalent to _____ inch(es).
5. A child was prescribed 1 fluidram of cough syrup, four times a day, as needed. The child's mother administered _____ teaspoon(s) each time the medication was given.

6. The nurse administered aspirin gr v. She knew this was equivalent to _____ milligram(s).

7. The nurse instilled 3 minims of Lacrisert into the patient's right eye, three times per day. The nurse knew that 3 minims was equal to _____ drop(s).

8. The physician prescribed 0.4 milligrams of atropine sulfate to be administered intramuscularly. The medication was labeled in grains/mL. The nurse knew to look for an ampule labeled _____ grains/mL.

9. A patient was to take 2 tablespoons of milk of magnesia. Because a medicine cup was available, he poured the milk of magnesia up to the _____ dram calibration line.

10. A 20-kg child was to receive Cosmegen, 15 mcg/kg of body weight. The child should receive _____ mcg or _____ mg.

11. A pregnant woman was prescribed 60 mg of Fergon daily. Her cumulative monthly dose (30 days) would be approximately _____ grams.

12. A patient who receives 3 teaspoons or 1 tablespoon of Kayexalate four times per day would be receiving a daily dose equivalent to _____ ounces.

13. A patient takes Aldomet, 500-mg tablets, three to four times per day. He is advised not to exceed a daily dose of 3 grams or _____ tablets.

14. A patient is to receive 250 mg of Ceclor, three times daily. The medicine is available in oral suspension, 250 mg per 5 mL. The nurse would give _____ teaspoon(s) or _____ dram(s).

15. An elderly patient is prescribed 30 mg of
    Elavil daily as a single bedtime dose. Elavil
    is available in syrup at a concentration of 10
    mg/5 mL. The nurse would give _____ mL
    or _____ teaspoons.

16. A patient is to receive 200 mg of Suprax
    every 12 hours. Because the tablet is
    available in 200-mg quantities, the patient
    would receive _____ gram(s) per day.

17. A child is prescribed 250 mg of Dynapen
    every 6 hours. The nurse gives two tablets,
    four times a day. Each tablet would be _____
    mg for a daily total dosage of _____ gram(s).

18. A renal patient, whose daily fluid intake is
    restricted to 1200 mL/day, is prescribed
    eight oral medications, three times daily.
    The nurse restricts the water needed for
    swallowing the medications so the patient
    can have fluids with his meals. The patient
    is allowed 5 ounces of water, three times a
    day with his medications. Therefore, the
    patient has _____ mL with his drugs.

Convert each item to its equivalent value.

1. 0.080 g = _____ mg

2. 3.2 liters = _____ mL

3. 1500 mcg = _____ mg

4. 0.125 mg = _____ mcg

5. 20 kg = _____ g

6. 5 mg = _____ g

7. ℥ ss̈ = _____ dram(s)

8. 30 minims = __ dram(s)

9. 15 grains = ___ dram(s)

10. 1/2 quart = _____ounces

11. 3 pints = _____ quart(s)

12. 8 drams = ____ ounce(s)

13. 1 tbs = _____ tsp

14. 6 tsp = _____ ounce(s)

15. 1 teacup = _____ounces

16. 2 tbs = _____ ounce(s)

17. gr ss̈ = _____mg

18. 30 grams = ___ ounce(s)

19. 1 oz = _____ mL

20. 1 gr = _____ mg

21. 3 tsp = _____mL

22. 20 kg = _____ pounds

23. gr 1/150 = _____mg

24. 0.3 mg = _____ gr

Dosage Calculation

Accurate dosage calculations are an essential component of the total nursing role in the safe administration of medications. Drugs are prescribed by their generic (official) name or trade (brand) names and are usually packaged in an average unit dosage. Tablets and capsules contain a solid concentration of drug (Tylenol gr x), whereas solutions contain a specific amount of drug (usually gram weight) dissolved in a specific amount of solution (usually milliliters or cc's) (Demerol at 50 mg per mL). Medication orders refer to drug dosages, so calculations will be necessary if a dosage prescribed is different from the available dosage.

Parenteral medications (IM, SC, IV) are packaged in vials, ampules, and premeasured syringes. Dosages usually range from 1 to 3 mL. Some drugs are measured in units (heparin, insulin, penicillin), and others are found in solutions as mEq (grams per 1 mL of solution). Some solutions need to be reconstituted from a powder form.

All medications come packaged and are clearly labeled. Some are available as a single dose, and others are available in multiple doses. Each label must contain specific information as outlined in Chapter 10. You should never prepare or administer any medication that is not clearly labeled.

Infants and children cannot receive the same dose of medication as adults. This is because a child's physiologic immaturity influences how a drug is absorbed, excreted, distributed, and used. Pediatric dosages are based on age, body weight, or body surface area. If you are going to be giving pediatric drugs, you must become familiar with the rules for calculating pediatric dosages. Refer to Appendix G for Nursing Concerns for Pediatric Drug Administration and Appendix H for Nursing Concerns for Geriatric Drug Administration.

This section will present common dosage calculations necessary for preparing for the oral and parenteral routes. See Appendix I for abbreviations used for drug preparation and administration.

10

Medication Labels

The accurate interpretation of a medication order and the drug label is the responsibility of the person preparing the medication. Medication labels contain a variety of information, depending on the complexity of the drug composition (eg, solid or liquid), drug availability (eg, tablets, vials, single-injection preparations), and dosage (eg, single or multiple doses, percentage strengths). Precautions about storage and protection from light can also be found on labels. Frequently the drug manufacturer encloses printed information about the drug.

To prepare the correct medication that is prescribed, you must be able to accurately read a drug label and be familiar with about 10 different key points or features. This chapter will present those features. Several drug labels will be depicted as examples, and sample drug problems will be presented.

⊕ READING A DRUG LABEL

All drug labels must contain specific drug information.

♦ **Drug name:** Medications are prescribed by their trade/brand or generic names. It is important to understand the differences. Most labels contain both names because drugs are ordered by either name.

Trade or brand name: The commercial name that the pharmaceutical company gives a drug. It is printed in bold, large, or capital letters on the label. The ® identifies manufacturer ownership. The drug may be manufactured by several companies, each using its own trade name.

Generic or official name: The chemical name of the drug as it is listed in the National Formulary. It appears in smaller letters, sometimes in parentheses. A drug has only one chemical name, used by all drug manufacturers, but it may have many different trade names.

♦ **Official national drug listings**

United States Pharmacopeia (USP)
National Formulary (NF)

- **Drug dosage and strength:** The dosage of the drug available for use in the container. Sometimes the dosage is expressed in two systems because the drug may be prescribed either way. For example, Synthroid may be prescribed as 50 mcg or 0.05 mg. Dosage strength is indicated in a solid form (grams, milligrams, milliequivalents, micrograms) in a solid form within a liquid (milliliters, teaspoons) or in other preparations such as ointments or patches.

- **Drug form:** The form in which the drug is prepared by the manufacturer, for example, tablets, capsules, injectables, oral suspensions, and ointments. Some drugs are prepared in several forms.

- **Drug quantity:** The amount of the drug in the container (100 tablets, 30 capsules, 10 mL) or the total amount of liquid available after reconstitution.

- **Drug administration:** The route indicated on the label, such as oral, sublingual, IM, IV, "by injection," or by "oral suspension."

IDENTIFYING THE COMPONENTS OF A DRUG LABEL

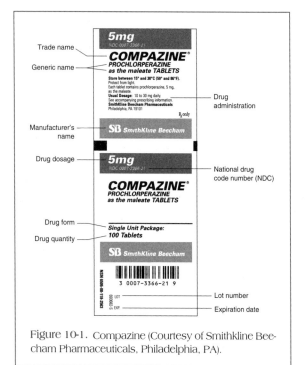

Figure 10-1. Compazine (Courtesy of Smithkline Beecham Pharmaceuticals, Philadelphia, PA).

➤ *PRACTICE PROBLEMS* ➤

Fill in the blanks for the following questions, referring to the medication label for Requip depicted in Figure 10-2.

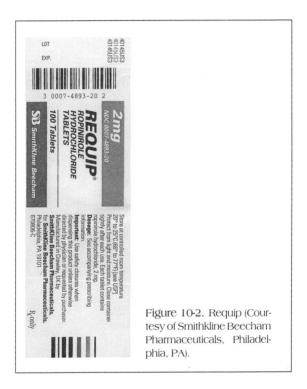

Figure 10-2. Requip (Courtesy of Smithkline Beecham Pharmaceuticals, Philadelphia, PA).

1. The generic name is _____.

2. The NDC number is _____.

3. The dosage strength is _____.

4. The drug quantity is _____.

5. The drug form is _____.

⊕ **INTERPRETING A DRUG LABEL**

Some labels are easy to read because they contain a limited amount of information, for example, labels for unit dose preparation where each tablet or capsule is separately packaged. This is the most common type of label that you will see in a hospital setting. Other labels indicate multiple tablets or capsules, with the dosage of each drug clearly visible.

Examine the drug label for multiple doses of Compazine (see Figure 10-1). Each of the 100 tablets contains 5 mg of the solid drug prochlorperazine. The usual dose of 10 mg to 30 mg per day means that a patient may receive 2 to 6 tablets daily.

Some solid preparations are available in a liquid solution. See Figure 10-3, which shows the drug label for Augmentin. When the powder is reconstituted with 47 mL of water, each 5 mL of liquid contains 200 mg of the drug.

Parenteral preparation labels will indicate dosages in a variety of ways: percentage and ratio strengths, milliequivalents (number of grams in 1 mL of a solution), 100 units per mL (insulin dosages), and powdered forms that have reconstitution directions. See Figure 10-4, which presents the drug label for Ancef. Each vial contains approximately 225 mg/mL after the addition of 2 mL of sterile water.

Frequently drugs are ordered in a unit of measure different than what is available. Mathematical conversions will be required, which will be covered in detail in the chapters that follow.

(text continues on page 128)

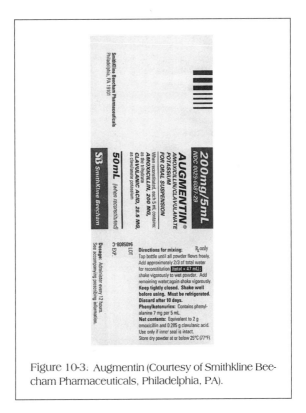

Figure 10-3: Augmentin (Courtesy of Smithkline Beecham Pharmaceuticals, Philadelphia, PA).

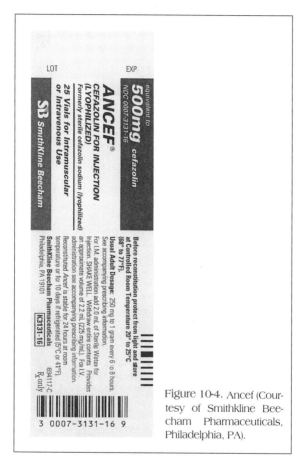

Figure 10-4. Ancef (Courtesy of Smithkline Beecham Pharmaceuticals, Philadelphia, PA).

END OF CHAPTER REVIEW

Answer each question by referring to the specific drug label presented in Figures 10-5, 10-6, 10-7, 10-8, and 10-9.

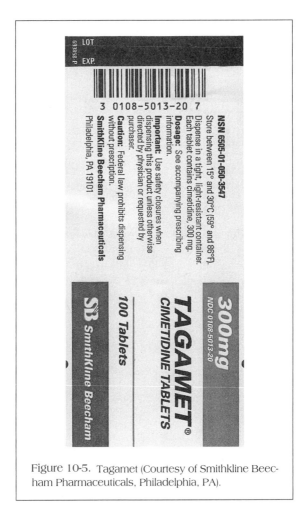

Figure 10-5. Tagamet (Courtesy of Smithkline Beecham Pharmaceuticals, Philadelphia, PA).

1. A physician prescribed 300 milligrams of Tagamet four times a day. The nurse would administer _____ tablet(s) for each dose. The patient would receive _____ milligrams of Tagamet in 24 hours.

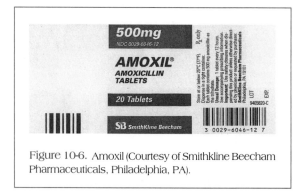

Figure 10-6. Amoxil (Courtesy of Smithkline Beecham
Pharmaceuticals, Philadelphia, PA).

2. A patient is to receive 2 grams of amoxicillin
   every 24 hours for 10 days. The medication is
   given every 6 hours. The patient would
   receive _____ milligrams or _____ grams for
   each dose.

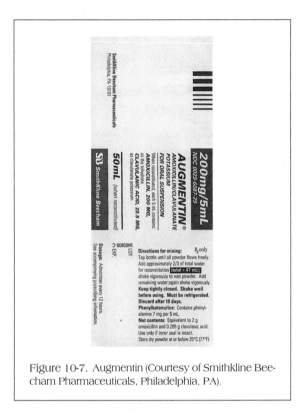

Figure 10-7. Augmentin (Courtesy of Smithkline Beecham Pharmaceuticals, Philadelphia, PA).

3. A physician prescribed 100 milligrams of Augmentin every 8 hours for a 3-year-old. The medication comes in a powder for an oral suspension, with a concentration of 200 mg/5 mL. The nurse would administer _____ mL for each dose. The child would receive _____ mg and _____ mL in 24 hours.

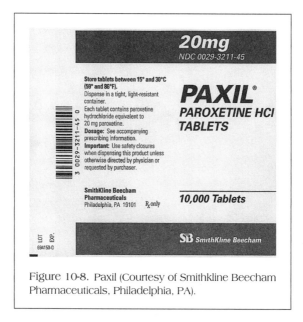

Figure 10-8. Paxil (Courtesy of Smithkline Beecham Pharmaceuticals, Philadelphia, PA).

4. A physician prescribed 20 milligrams of Paxil twice a day. The patient would receive _____ tablet(s) per dose and _____ milligrams per day.

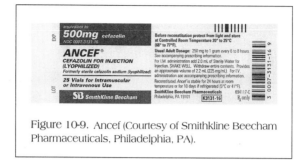

Figure 10-9. Ancef (Courtesy of Smithkline Beecham Pharmaceuticals, Philadelphia, PA).

5. A physician prescribed 1 gram of Ancef, intravenously, every 8 hours. The nurse would need to mix _____ vial(s) for each dose.

6. A patient is prescribed 500 mg of Ancef intramuscularly, immediately. The nurse would reconstitute the vial of Ancef with _____ mL of sterile water for injection.

11

Oral Dosage Calculations

The oral route is a simple, economic method of drug delivery that is safe and convenient for the systemic administration of medications. Most tablets, capsules, and Caplets come in the dosage prescribed, or the prescription requires giving more than one pill or dividing a scored tablet in half. Capsules, Caplets, and enteric-coated tablets should not be broken in half.

When the prescribed or desired dosage is different from what is available or what "you have," a dosage calculation is necessary to determine the quantity of drug to give. Use ratios and proportions, presented in Chapter 5, to solve the dosage calculations.

An alternate method to ratios and proportions that can be used to quickly solve dosage problems is use of the *Formula Method.* The *Formula Method* is very easy when calculating dosages *in the same system* and the *same units of measurement.* The symbol ℞ is used throughout to indicate the desired amount.

⊕ USE OF RATIOS AND PROPORTIONS: SOLVING FOR *X*

Frequently a physician prescribes a medication in a quantity that is different than the amount or quantity available. The difference in the dosage can be for medications in the same system (eg, 0.250 mg of digoxin prescribed and 0.125 mg of digoxin available) or for medications in different systems (eg, 0.8 grams of Anturan is prescribed, and the drug is available in grains). When determining the *unknown quantity,* you need to *solve for x,* using the ratio and proportion format (presented on pages 71–77) or use the abbreviated Formula Method explained here.

⊕ FORMULA METHOD

$$\frac{\text{D (desired amount)}}{\text{H (have available)}} \times \text{Q (quantity)}$$

$$= x \text{ (amount to give)}$$

$$\left[\frac{\text{D}}{\text{H}} \times \text{Q} = x \right]$$

⊕ DOSAGE PROBLEMS FOR MEDICATIONS IN THE SAME SYSTEM

EXAMPLE:　R̶:　　0.250 mg digoxin
　　　　Have:　0.125 mg digoxin/tablet
　　　　Give:　＿＿＿ tablet(s)

Use: $$\frac{D}{H} \times Q = x$$

$$\frac{0.250 \text{ mg}}{0.125 \text{ mg}} = 0.250 \div 0.125 = 2$$

$2 \times (1 \text{ tablet}) = 2$

Answer = 2 tablets

EXAMPLE: ℞:   gr 1/2 of codeine sulfate, p.r.n.
Have: gr 1/4/tablet
Give: _____ tablet(s)

Use: $$\frac{D}{H} \times Q = x$$

$$\frac{\text{gr } 1/2}{\text{gr } 1/4} = \frac{1}{\mathbf{2}_1} \times \frac{\mathbf{4}^2}{1} = \frac{2}{1} = 2$$

$2 \times (1 \text{ tablet}) = 2$

Answer = 2 tablets

EXAMPLE: ℞:   100 mg of phenobarbital elixir
Have: 20 mg/5mL
Give: _____ mL

Use: $$\frac{D}{H} \times Q = x$$

$$\frac{100 \text{ mg}}{20 \text{ mg}} = 100 \div 20 = 5$$

$5 \times (5 \text{ mL}) = 25$

Answer = 25 mL

DOSAGE PROBLEMS FOR MEDICATIONS IN THE SAME SYSTEM BUT HAVING DIFFERENT UNITS OF MEASUREMENT

Sometimes dosages are prescribed in *different units of measurement within the same system.* Then you need to *convert* them to like units. It is best to change the dosage to the smaller unit to avoid the use of decimals or fractions.

EXAMPLE:	℞:	4 grams of Gantrisin, q.i.d.
	Have:	500 mg/tablet
	Give:	_____ tablet(s)

Convert to Like Units: To convert 4 g to mg, move the decimal point (4.0 g) three places to the right: 4.000. ↖

Then 4 g = 4000 mg

Use:

$$\frac{D}{H} \times Q = x$$

$$\frac{4,000 \text{ mg}}{500 \text{ mg}} = \frac{4000}{500} = \frac{40}{5} = 8$$

Answer = 8 tablets

EXAMPLE:	℞:	1.2 grams of Equanil in 2 divided doses
	Have:	600 mg/tablet
	Give:	_____ tablet(s)

Convert   To convert 1.2 g to mg, move the
to Like   decimal point (1.2 g) three places to
Units: the right: 1.200. ↖

Then 1.2 g = 1200 mg

Use: $\dfrac{D}{H} \times Q = x$

$\dfrac{1200 \text{ mg}}{600 \text{ mg}} = 1200 \div 600 = 2$

$2 \times$ quantity (1 tablet) = 2

Answer = 2 tablets in 2 divided doses
or 1 tablet each dose

➤ *PRACTICE PROBLEMS* ➤

1. Furosemide (Lasix) 160 mg daily is
   prescribed. Lasix 40-mg tablets are on hand.
   Give _____ tablet(s).

2. Trilisate 1500 mg is prescribed. Trilisate liquid
   is labeled 500 mg per 5 mL. Give _____ mL.

3. Allopurinol 150 mg is prescribed. Allopurinol
   300-mg tablets are on hand. Give _____
   tablet(s).

4. Codeine elixir 20 mg is prescribed. Codeine
   elixir is labeled 10 mg per 5 mL. Give _____
   mL.

5. Brethine 7.5 mg t.i.d. is prescribed. Brethine
   2.5-mg tablets are on hand. Give _____
   tablet(s), t.i.d.

6. Demerol 100 mg is to be taken every 4 to 6 hours, as needed. Demerol 50-mg tablets are on hand. Give _____ tablet(s) for each dose.

7. Phenobarbital elixir 75 mg is prescribed. Phenobarbital elixir is labeled 15 mg/mL. Give _____ mL.

8. HydroDIURIL 25 mg is prescribed. HydroDIURIL 50-mg tablets are on hand. Give _____ tablet(s).

9. Synthroid 0.030 mg is prescribed. Synthroid 0.05-mg tablets are on hand. Give _____ tablet(s).

10. Coumadin 10 mg is prescribed. Coumadin 2.5-mg tablets are on hand. Give _____ tablet(s).

11. Mellaril 75 mg is prescribed t.i.d. Mellaril 25-mg tablets are on hand. Give _____ tablet(s).

12. Dilantin 300 mg is prescribed. Dilantin suspension is labeled 125 mg per 5 mL. Give _____ mL.

13. Depakene 0.75 grams is prescribed. Depakene syrup is labeled 250 mg per 5 mL. Give _____ mL.

14. Zarontin syrup 0.5 grams is prescribed. Zarontin syrup is labeled 250 mg per 5 mL. Give _____ mL.

15. Azulfidine 4 grams is to be taken in four equally divided portions. Azulfidine 500-mg tablets are on hand. Give _____ tablet(s) each dose.

16. Choledyl 0.25 g is prescribed. Choledyl elixir is labeled 100 mg per 5 mL. Give _____ mL.

17. Robicillin VK 2.0 grams daily is prescribed. Robicillin VK 250-mg tablets are on hand. Give _____ tablet(s) each day.

18. Amoxicillin 0.5 g every 8 hours is prescribed. Amoxicillin oral suspension is labeled 250 mg/teaspoon. Give _____ mL.

19. Tigan 0.30 grams daily is prescribed. Tigan 100-mg capsules are on hand. Give _____ tablet(s) each day.

20. Provera 10 mg is prescribed. Provera 2.5-mg tablets are on hand. Give _____ tablet(s).

21. Motrin 0.8 g is prescribed. Motrin 400-mg tablets are on hand. Give _____ tablet(s).

✚ DOSAGE PROBLEMS FOR MEDICATIONS IN DIFFERENT SYSTEMS

> ➤ RULE: Whenever the desired and available drug doses are in different systems, you would perform the following steps:

1. Choose the approximate equivalent and convert both to the same system. Choose the system that you have available.
2. Use ratio and proportion to solve for x.
3. Use the formula D/H $\times$ Q = x if possible.

EXAMPLE: ℞:   0.8 grams of a drug daily
                 Give: _____ grains daily

Convert to   Grains are *available.* Change 0.8 g
Same   to gr.
System:
Equivalent: 1 gram = 15 grains

Complete   1 gram: 15 grains :: 0.8 grams : *x* grains
the   1 × *x* = 0.8 × 15
Proportion:

Solve for x: 1*x* = 12

                                Answer = 12 grains or gr xii

EXAMPLE: ℞:   45 cc Elixophyllin elixir
                 Give: _____ fluidrams

Convert to   Fluidrams are *available.* Change 45
Same   cc's to f℥.
System:
Equivalent: 30 cc = 8 f℥

Complete   30 cc : 8 f℥ :: 45 cc : *x* f℥
the
Proportion: 30 × *x* = 45 × 8

Solve for x: 30*x* = 45 × 8

                30*x* = 360

                $$\frac{30x}{30} = \frac{360}{30}$$

                $$x = \frac{360}{30} = 360 \div 30 = 12$$

Reduce: $x = 12$ f3

$$Answer = 12 \text{ f3 or f3xii}$$

EXAMPLE: R: Morphine sulfate grain 1/4
               Have: Morphine sulfate 10-mg tablets
               Give: _____ tablet(s)

Convert to   Milligrams are *available.*
Same   Change gr 1/4 to mg
System:
Equivalent: 1 grain = 60 mg

Complete   1 grain : 60 mg :: 1/4 grain : x mg
the
Proportion:

$$1 \times x = \frac{1}{4} \times 60$$

Solve for x: $1x = \dfrac{1}{4} \times 60$

$$1x = 15$$
$$x = 15 \text{ mg}$$

Use: $$\frac{D}{H} \times Q = x$$

$$\frac{15 \text{ mg}}{10 \text{ mg}} = 15 \div 10 = 1.5$$

$$1.5 \times 1 \text{ tablet}$$

$$= 1.5 \text{ or } 1\frac{1}{2} \text{ tablets}$$

$$Answer = 1\frac{1}{2} \text{ tablets}$$

PRACTICE PROBLEMS

1. Thorazine hydrochloride is on hand in syrup (2 mg/mL). The prescribed dose is 3 teaspoons. Give _____ mL, which would be equal to _____ mg.

2. Mysoline is on hand in a liquid as 250 mg/5 mL. The initial dose of 125 mg for 3 days requires giving _____ teaspoon(s) each day for a total of _____ mL over 3 days.

3. Scopolamine hydrobromide is on hand in a transdermal patch containing 0.0015 grams. The system delivers 0.5 mg over 72 hours. After 72 hours, grains _____ remain.

4. Tylenol gr x is prescribed. Tylenol elixir is labeled 160 mg per teaspoon. Give _____ mL.

5. Colchicine 1.2 mg is prescribed. Colchicine gr 1/100 is on hand. Give _____ tablet(s).

6. Zaroxolyn is on hand in gr 1/6 tablets. The prescribed dose is 20 mg. Give _____ tablet(s).

7. Potassium chloride gr v is prescribed. Potassium chloride 300-mg tablets are available. Give _____ tablet(s).

8. Vistaril 50-mg oral suspension is ordered. Vistaril is available as 25 mg/5 mL. Give _____ teaspoons.

9. Nitroglycerin tablets gr 1/100 are prescribed. Available are 0.6-mg tablets. Give _____ tablet(s).

10. Ceclor oral suspension 500 mg is prescribed. Ceclor is available as 250 mg/5 mL. Give _____ mL = _____ teaspoons.

11. Kay Ciel (potassium chloride) 20 mEq, q.i.d. is prescribed. Kay Ciel elixir is available as 6.7 mEq/5 mL. Give _____ mL or _____ ounce(s).

12. Nembutal gr i s̄s̄ is prescribed. The drug is available in 50-mg capsules. Give _____ capsule(s). The dose is approximate.

⊕ PEDIATRIC DOSAGES

RULES BASED ON AGE

> ► FRIED'S RULE: To determine dosage for newborns to 2-year-olds, perform the following steps:

♦ Determine the child's age in months.
♦ Divide the age in months by 150.
♦ Multiply by the adult dose.
♦ Use $\dfrac{\text{age in months}}{150} \times$ normal adult dose.
♦ If necessary, use $\dfrac{\text{desired amount}}{\text{amount on hand}} \times$ quantity = amount to give.

EXAMPLE: The physician prescribed Dolanex elixir for a 15-month-old. The normal adult dose is 325 mg every 4 to 6 hours. Dolanex elixir is available as 325 mg/5 mL.

Use Fried's Rule:

$$\text{Pediatric dose} = \frac{\text{age in months}}{150}$$

$\times$ normal adult dose

$$\text{Pediatric dose} = \frac{15 \text{ months}}{150}$$

$$= \frac{1}{10} \times 325 \text{ mg} = 32.5 \text{ mg}$$

Because Dolanex is available as 325 mg/5 mL, additional computation is necessary to determine the amount of milliliters to give.

Use:

$$\frac{D}{H} \times Q = x$$

$= $ amount to give

$$\frac{32.5 \text{ mg}}{325} = \frac{1}{10}$$

$$\frac{1}{10} \times 5.0 \text{ mL} = 0.5 \text{ mL}$$

Answer $= 0.5$ mL

> ▶ YOUNG'S RULE: To determine dosage for children ages 1 to 12, perform the following steps:

- Determine the child's age in years.
- Divide the age in years by the age in years + 12.
- Multiply by the adult dose.
- Use $\dfrac{\text{age (in years)}}{\text{age (in years)} + 12} \times$ normal adult dose.

• If necessary, use $\dfrac{\text{desired amount}}{\text{amount on hand}} \times$ quantity

= amount to give.

EXAMPLE: The physician prescribed milk of magnesia for an 8-year-old patient. The normal adult dose is 30 mL.

Use Young's Rule: Pediatric dose = $\dfrac{\text{age (in years)}}{\text{age (in years)} + 12}$

$\times$ normal adult dose

Pediatric dose = $\dfrac{8}{8 + 12}$

$= \dfrac{8}{20} = \dfrac{2}{\cancel{5}_1} \times \cancel{30}_6 \text{ mL} = 12 \text{ mL}$

Answer = 12 mL

EXAMPLE: A physician prescribed Dolanex elixir for a 4-year-old. The normal adult dose is 325 mg every 4 to 6 hours. Dolanex elixir is available as 325 mg/5 mL.

Use Young's Rule: Pediatric dose = $\dfrac{\text{age (in years)}}{\text{age (in years)} + 12}$

$\times$ normal adult dose

Pediatric dose = $\dfrac{4}{4 + 12} = \dfrac{4}{16}$

$$= \frac{1}{4} \times 325 \text{ mg} = 81 \text{ mg}$$

Use: $\frac{\text{D}}{\text{H}} \times \text{Q} = x$

= amount to give

$$\frac{81 \text{ mg}}{325} = \frac{1}{4} \text{ (approximate)}$$

$$\frac{1}{4} \times 5.0 \text{ mL} = 1.25 \text{ mL}$$

Answer = 1.25 mL

RULES BASED ON WEIGHT

> ► CLARK'S RULE: To determine dosage for 2-year-olds and older children, perform the following steps:

- ◆ Determine the child's weight in pounds.
- ◆ Divide the weight by 150.
- ◆ Multiply by the normal adult dose.

- ◆ Use $\dfrac{\text{weight in pounds}}{150} \times$ normal adult dose.

- ◆ If necessary, use $\dfrac{\text{desired amount}}{\text{amount on hand}} \times$ quantity

= amount to give.

EXAMPLE: The physician prescribed Dolanex elixir for a 4-year-old who weighs about 30 pounds. The normal adult dose is 325 mg every 4 to 6 hours. Dolanex elixir is available as 325 mg/5 mL.

Use Clark's Rule:

$$\text{Pediatric dose} = \frac{\text{weight in pounds}}{150}$$

$$\times \text{ normal adult dose}$$

$$\text{Pediatric dose} = \frac{30}{150} = \frac{1}{5}$$

$$\frac{1}{5} \times 325 \text{ mg} = 65 \text{ mg}$$

Use:

$$\frac{D}{H} \times Q = x$$

$$= \text{amount to give}$$

$$\frac{65}{325} = \frac{1}{5}$$

$$\frac{1}{5} \times 5 \text{ mL} = 1.0 \text{ mL}$$

Answer = 1.0 mL

Sometimes medications are prescribed in milligrams/kilogram of body weight. Because there are 2.2 pounds in a kilogram, you must convert the child's weight in pounds to kilograms before you can calculate the drug dosage. The following rule tells you how to calculate drug dosages when the drug is ordered according to kilograms of body weight.

> ➤ RULE: To change pounds to kilograms, follow these steps:

- Determine the patient's body weight in pounds.
- Divide by 2.2.
- Solve the problem using the appropriate rule.

EXAMPLE: The physician prescribed 20 mg of amoxicillin/kg of body weight to be administered q 8 hours in equally divided doses. The patient weighed 44 pounds and was 5 years old. Divide by 2.2 to determine body weight in kilograms.

Move the decimal point in the divisor and the dividend the same number of places. Put the decimal point directly above the line for the quotient.

$$2.2. \quad \overline{)44.0.}$$

$$\begin{array}{r} 20. \text{ (quotient)} \\ 22\overline{)440.} \end{array}$$

Answer = 20 kg

Use: Use a proportion to solve for x.

20 mg : 1 kg :: x mg : 20 kg

$1x = 20 \times 20$

$1x = 400$

$x = 400$ mg

400 mg will be divided into three
equal doses. 400 mg ÷ 3 = 133 mg to
be given every 8 hours.

Answer = 133 mg

RULE BASED ON BODY SURFACE AREA

Basing a pediatric dosage on body surface area is
the most accurate way of determining the amount
of drug to give.

> ➤ RULE: To determine a pediatric dosage
> based on body surface area, perform the
> following steps:

+ Estimate the child's body surface area in
  square meters (m²). Refer to a nomogram
  (Figure 11-1).*
+ Use

  $$\frac{\text{child's surface area in square meters}}{1.73 \text{ m}^2 \text{ (surface area of an average adult)}}$$

  × adult dose.
+ If necessary, use a proportion to solve for *x*.

---

*The nomogram is used to determine body surface
area. To use the nomograms in Figure 11-1, you
need to draw a straight line from the patient's
height to his or her weight. You will intersect the
surface area column at a number that indicates the
patient's body surface area in square meters (m²).

EXAMPLE: The physician prescribed Benadryl
150 mg/m²/day for an 8-year-old child
who weighs 75 pounds and is 50
inches tall (4 feet, 2 inches). The normal adult dose is 25 mg QID. The
nurse would give _____ mg QID.

Use Body Surface Area Rule:

$$\frac{\text{child's surface area in square meters (m}^2)}{1.73 \text{ m}^2}$$

× adult dose

$$\frac{1.05 \text{ m}^2}{1.73} = 0.60 \times 25 \text{ mg} = 15.17 \text{ mg}$$

To prepare Benadryl for administration, it would be best to
drop the .17 and prepare 15 mg.

Answer = 15 mg, QID.

(text continues on page 154)

**Nomogram for Estimating the Surface Area of Infants
and Young Children**

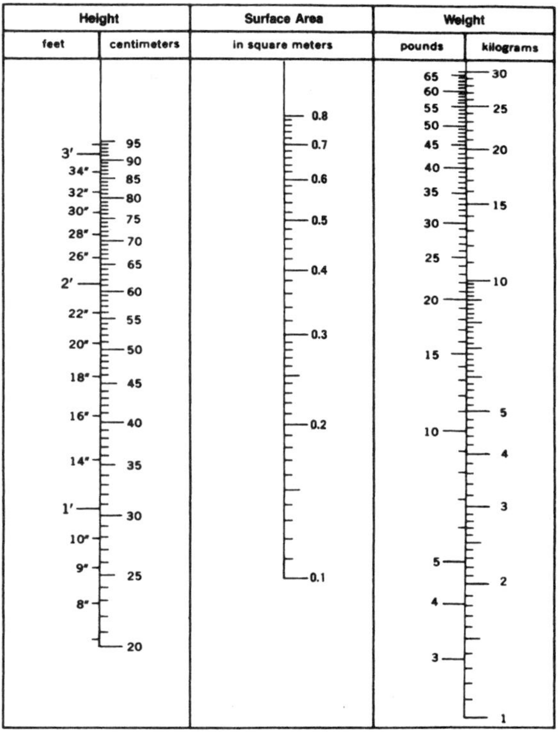

Figure 11-1. Nomograms for estimating surface area of body. Nomogram on opposite page indicates 1.05m² surface area for a child who weighs 75 pounds and is 4 feet, 2 inches tall. (Illustrations courtesy of Abbott Laboratories, North Chicago, IL.)

**Nomogram for Estimating the Surface Area
of Older Children and Adults**

Height		Surface Area	Weight	
feet	centimeters	in square meters	pounds	kilograms

END OF CHAPTER REVIEW

Solve the following problems:

1. Coumadin sodium 30 mg daily is prescribed. Coumadin sodium 10-mg tablets are on hand. Give _____ tablet(s).

2. Ascorbic acid 300 mg is prescribed. Ascorbic acid 100-mg tablets are on hand. Give _____ tablet(s).

3. Mysoline 1.5 grams daily is prescribed. Mysoline liquid is labeled 250 mg per 5 mL. Give _____ mL.

4. HydroDIURIL 0.2 grams is prescribed. HydroDIURIL 50-mg tablets are on hand. Give _____ tablet(s).

5. Atropine sulfate is on hand in 0.3-mg tablets. The prescribed dose is grain 1/200. Give _____ tablet(s).

6. Serax is available in 15-mg tablets. The prescribed daily dose is grains 1/2. Give _____ tablet(s).

7. Cepulac 20 grams is prescribed. Cephulac 30 grams in 45 mL is on hand. Give _____ ounce(s).

8. Nitroglycerin grains 1/150 is prescribed. Nitroglycerin 0.4-mg tablets are on hand. Give _____ tablet(s).

9. Morphine sulfate grains 1/4 is prescribed. Morphine sulfate oral solution is labeled 10 mg per 5 mL. Give _____ mL.

10. Darvocet-N 0.1 gram is prescribed. Darvocet-N is on hand as 100-mg tablets. Give _____ tablet(s).

11. Nardil gr 1/4 four times a day is prescribed. Nardil is on hand in 15-mg tablets. Give _____ tablet(s) per dose for a total of _____ tablet(s) daily.

12. Anavar 10 mg daily for 2 weeks is prescribed. Anavar is available in 2.5-mg tablets. Give _____ tablets daily, equally divided over 6 hours.

13. DiaBeta 5 mg is prescribed. DiaBeta is on hand in 1.25-mg tablets. Give _____ tablet(s).

14. Nystatin oral suspension, 500,000 units, q.i.d. was prescribed. Nystatin is on hand as 100,000 U/mL. Give _____ teaspoon(s) or _____ dram(s).

15. Erythromycin 500 mg is prescribed. Erythromycin is on hand as 0.25 g/5 mL. Give _____ mL or _____ teaspoon(s).

16. The physician prescribed Capoten, 1.5 grams daily in three equal doses, for hypertension. The nurse would give _____ -mg tablet(s), three times a day.

17. The physician prescribed Nalfon 2.4 grams daily for rheumatoid arthritis. The tablets are available as 600 mg. The nurse would give _____ tablet(s) a day.

18. Phenobarbital 30 mg was ordered. Tablets are available as gr 1/4. The nurse would give _____ tablet(s).

19. Potassium chloride tablets are available in 300-mg doses. The physician prescribed gr v. Give _____ tablet(s).

20. The physician prescribed Spectrobid 25 mg/kg for a 22-pound 12-month-old. The medicine was to be given q12h. The child would receive _____ mg every 12 hours.

21. A physician prescribed Pen-Vee K for an 18-month-old. The medicine comes in a powder for oral suspension, 250 mg/5 mL. The normal adult dose is 250 mg every 6 hours. The nurse would give _____ mg in _____ mL every 6 hours.

22. The physician prescribed Benadryl for an 8-year-old to relieve itching from chicken pox. Benadryl comes in an elixir of 12.5 mg/5 mL. The normal adult dose is 25 mg every 12 hours as needed. The nurse would give _____ mg in _____ mL every 12 hours.

23. A physician prescribed Dimetane for a 30-pound 4-year-old. The drug comes as an elixir, 2 mg/5 mL. The normal adult dose is 4.0 mg every 4 to 6 hours. The nurse would give _____ mg in _____ mL every 4 to 6 hours.

24. A physician prescribed Phenergan for a 45-pound child for preoperative medication. Phenergan is to be given as 1 mg/kg of body weight. The nurse would give _____ mg preoperatively.

25. A physician prescribed Pelamine for a 7-year-old who weighs 70 pounds and is 50 inches tall. The drug is to be administered as 150 mg/m^2 day in four equal doses. The normal adult dose is 50 mg every 6 hours. Refer to the nomogram in Figure 11–1 to find the child's surface area in square meters. Calculate the dosage the child should receive in four equally divided doses. _____

Parenteral Dosages

The term *parenteral* refers to any route of drug delivery other than the digestive tract (enteral route). Parenteral commonly refers to the injection of drugs into body tissues (using a needle and syringe) and into body fluids. *Needle precautions should always be followed.* Parenteral drugs must be sterile and should absorb easily without causing tissue irritation.

The parenteral route is recommended if a medication would be ineffectively absorbed in the gastrointestinal tract or take too long to become effective. Parenteral drugs are administered in the form of sterile liquid preparations.

Drugs for injection are most commonly supplied in liquid form in ampules or vials and are given in a 3-cc syringe; quantities <1 mL can be given in a tuberculin syringe (see Figure 12-1). Insulin syringes are presented in Chapter 14.

Pediatric parenteral medications are most commonly given via the subcutaneous and intramuscular routes. Dosage amount is limited to 1 mL per site for those under 5 years old, and dosages are usually measured using a tuberculin syringe. Refer to Appendix C for information on subcuta-

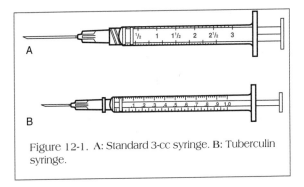

Figure 12-1. A: Standard 3-cc syringe. B: Tuberculin syringe.

neous injections and Appendix F for pediatric intramuscular injections. Chapter 15 covers immunostimulants, and Appendix G covers Nursing Concerns for Pediatric Drug Administration.

Dosage calculations can be solved by using ratios and proportions and/or by using the following formula:

$$\frac{\text{D (desired amount)}}{\text{H (have available)}} \times \text{Q (quantity)}$$

$$= x \text{ (amount to give)}$$

$$\left[\frac{\text{D}}{\text{H}} \times \text{Q} = x\right]$$

If you wish to review information about the different parenteral routes, please refer to Appendices B through E. Although this material is not specifically math related, it has been included for your convenience.

DOSAGE PROBLEMS FOR MEDICATIONS IN THE SAME SYSTEM BUT HAVING DIFFERENT UNITS OF MEASUREMENT*

EXAMPLE: $\mathbb{R}$:   1.0 mg folic acid
             Have: 5.0 mg/mL folic acid
             Give: _____ mL

Use: $\dfrac{D}{H} \times Q = x$

             $\dfrac{1.0 \text{ mg}}{5.0 \text{ mg}} = \dfrac{1}{5}$

             $\dfrac{1}{5} \times 1 \text{ mL} = 0.20 \text{ mL}$

                                    Answer = 0.20 mL

EXAMPLE: $\mathbb{R}$:   300 mg clindamycin
             Have: 150 mg/mL clindamycin
             Give: _____ mL

Use: $\dfrac{D}{H} \times Q = x$

             $\dfrac{300 \text{ mg}}{150 \text{ mg}} = \dfrac{2}{1}$

             $\dfrac{2}{1} \times 1 \text{ mL} = 2 \text{ mL}$

                                    Answer = 2 mL

---

*See pages 137–138 for directions.

EXAMPLE: ℞:   35 mg Demerol
                Have: 50 mg/mL
                Give: _____ mL

Use: $\dfrac{D}{H} \times Q = x$

                $\dfrac{35 \text{ mg}}{50 \text{ mg}} = \dfrac{7}{10}$

                $\dfrac{7}{10} \times$ quantity (1 mL) = 0.7 mL

                                Answer = 0.7 mL

EXAMPLE: ℞:   0.25 mg of Lanoxin
                Have: 500 mcg/2 mL
                Give: _____ mL

Convert   To convert 0.25 mg to mcg, move the
to Like   decimal point (0.25 mg) three places
Units: to the right 0.250. Then 0.25 mg =
                250 mcg.

Use: $\dfrac{D}{H} \times Q = x$

                $\dfrac{250 \text{ mcg}}{500 \text{ mcg}} = \dfrac{1}{2}$

                $\dfrac{1}{2} \times$ quantity (2 mL) = 1 mL

                                Answer = 1 mL

✣ DOSAGE PROBLEMS FOR MEDICATIONS IN DIFFERENT SYSTEMS

> ➤ RULE: Whenever the desired and available drug dosages are in different systems, you would perform the following steps:

1. Choose the approximate equivalent and convert both to the same system. Choose the system that you have available.
2. Use ratios and proportions to solve for x.
3. Use the formula D/H × Q = x if possible.

EXAMPLE: ℞:   gr iss of Garamycin IM, b.i.d.
              Have: Garamycin 60 mg per mL
              Give: _____ mL, b.i.d.

Equivalent: 1 grain = 60 milligrams

Complete the Proportion:

1 grain : 60 mg :: $1\frac{1}{2}$ grains : x mg

$1 \times x = 1\frac{1}{2} \times 60$

Solve for x:

$1x = 1\frac{1}{2} \times 60$

$1x = \dfrac{3}{\cancel{2}_1} \times \cancel{60}^{30}$

$x = 90$ mg

Use:

$$\frac{D}{H} \times Q = x$$

$$\frac{90 \text{ mg}}{60 \text{ mg}} = \frac{3}{2}$$

$$\frac{3}{2} \times 1 \text{ mL} = 1\frac{1}{2} \text{ mL}$$

$$Answer = 1\frac{1}{2} \text{ mL}$$

✦ MEDICATIONS PACKAGED AS POWDERS

Some drugs are unstable in solution so they are packaged as a powder. When the *available amount of drug* is in a solute form (dry powder), the drug needs to be reconstituted by adding a diluent (solvent). The label on the available drug will give directions for adding the diluent. There are three common diluents that must always be sterile when added to the dry powder. Use one of these three:

- Bacteriostatic water
- Sodium chloride (0.9%)
- Sterile water

Read labeled directions for reconstitution:

- Recommended diluent
- Quantity of diluent
- Ratio of solute to solvent after reconstitution

Use: $\dfrac{D}{H} \times Q = x$

After reconstitution:

+ Label medication with the date and time of preparation and expiration.
+ Initial the label.
+ *Remember:* Reconstituted solutions will always exceed the volume of the added diluent.

⊕ PREPARATION OF A SINGLE-STRENGTH SOLUTION

EXAMPLE: ℞: 250 mg of Ancef, IM, every 8 hours. The medication is available as a powder in a 1-gram vial.

Reconstitute: Labeled directions: Reconstitute by adding 2.5 mL of sterile water for injection. Shake well until dissolved. Solution concentration will equal 330 mg per mL. Fluid volume will equal 3.0 mL.

Dissolve 1 gram of powder with 2.5 mL of sterile water.

Use: $$\frac{D}{H} \times Q = x$$

$$\frac{250 \text{ mg}}{*1000 \text{ mg}} = \frac{1}{4}$$

$$\frac{1}{4} \times 3.0 \text{ mL} = 0.75 \text{ mL or } \frac{3}{4}$$

$$Answer = \frac{3}{4} \text{ mL}$$

---

*Approximate measure: 330 mg/1.0 mL = 990 mg/3.0 mL.

EXAMPLE: R: 125 mg of Solu-Medrol, IM. Medication is available as a powder in a 500-mg vial.

Reconstitute: Labeled directions: Reconstitute by adding 8 mL of sterile water for injection. Solution concentration will equal 62.5 mg per mL. Fluid volume will equal > 8 mL.

Dissolve 500 mg of powder with 8 mL of sterile water.

Use: $\dfrac{D}{H} \times Q = x$

$$\frac{125 \text{ mg}}{500 \text{ mg}} = \frac{1}{4} \times 8 \text{ mL} = 2 \text{ mL}$$

Answer = 2 mL

PREPARATION OF A MULTIPLE-STRENGTH SOLUTION

EXAMPLE: R: Geopen 1 g, IM. Medication is available as a powder in a 2-g vial.

Reconstitute: Labeled directions: Reconstitute by adding 4 mL of sterile water for IM injection (8 mL is required for IV use). Solution concentration (g/mL) will vary with mL of diluent added.

For example:

4 mL of diluent = 1 g/2.5 mL
5 mL of diluent = 1 g/3 mL
7.2 mL of diluent = 1 g/4 mL

Use: $\dfrac{\text{D}}{\text{H}} = \dfrac{1\text{g}}{1\ \text{g}/2.5\ \text{mL}}$

Answer = 2.5 mL

➤ PRACTICE PROBLEMS ➤

Complete the following problems by using the ratio and proportion and/or the Formula method:

1. The physician requested that a patient receive 0.002 grams of folic acid, IM, per day, for 5 days, for severe intestinal malabsorption. The injection was on hand as 1.0 mg/mL. The nurse would give _____ mL a day for 5 days.

2. The physician requested that 120 mg of furosemide be administered IM in three equally divided doses every 8 hours for 2 days. The drug is available for injection as 10 mg/mL. The nurse should give _____ mL every 8 hours.

3. Robaxin 0.3 grams, IM, was prescribed. The drug is available as 100 mg/mL for injection. The nurse would give _____ mL.

4. Compazine 15 mg, IM, is prescribed for severe nausea and vomiting. Compazine is available as 5 mg/mL. The nurse should give _____ mL.

5. Haldol 4 mg, IM, was prescribed. Haldol is available as 5 mg/mL. The nurse should give _____ mL.

END OF CHAPTER REVIEW

Complete the following problems by using the ratio and proportion and/or the Formula method:

1. Aldomet 125 mg was prescribed, IM, q.i.d. The medication was available for injection as 250 mg/5 mL. The nurse would administer _____ mL, q.i.d.

2. Valium 2 mg was prescribed, IM, p.r.n., every 3 to 4 hours. The medication was available for injection as 5 mg/mL. The nurse would give _____ mL every 3 to 4 hours as needed.

3. The physician requested that a patient receive 1.5 mg of Stadol, IM, every 3 to 4 hours as needed for pain. The medication was available for injection as 2.0 mg/mL. The nurse would give _____ mL every 3 to 4 hours, p.r.n.

4. Demerol 35 mg, IM, is prescribed for pain. Demerol was available for injection as 50 mg/mL. The nurse would give _____ mL.

5. The physician prescribed 6 mg of Aqua-MEPHYTON, IM, weekly. The medication was available as 2 mg/mL. The nurse would give _____ mL every week.

6. Versed 3 mg, IM, is prescribed preoperatively to induce drowsiness. Versed was available as 5 mg/mL. The nurse would give _____ mL.

7. The physician prescribed Dilaudid 3 mg, IM, every 4 to 6 hours for analgesia. Dilaudid is available as 4 mg/mL. The nurse would give _____ mL every 4 to 6 hours.

8. Lasix 30 mg, IM, is prescribed as a diuretic. Lasix was available as 40 mg/mL. The nurse would give _____ mL.

9. Atropine 0.5 mg was ordered preoperatively, to be given subcutaneously. The medication was available in a vial as grains 1/150 per 1.0 mL. The nurse would give _____ mL.

10. Scopolamine 0.3 mg was ordered subcutaneously as a preanesthetic medication. The medication was available in ampules containing grains 1/200 per mL. The nurse would give _____ mL.

11. The physician prescribed morphine sulfate grains 1/5, IM, every 4 to 6 hours for severe pain. The medication is available as 15 mg/mL. The nurse would give _____ mL, every 4 to 6 hours, as needed.

12. The physician prescribed grains iii of Seconal, IM. The medication is available as 100 mg/mL for injection. The nurse would give _____ mL.

13. Robinul 0.15 mg was ordered for gastrointestinal distress. Robinul is available as 0.2 mg/mL. The nurse would give _____ mL.

14. Vistaril 25 mg, IM, was ordered preoperatively. Vistaril is available as 100 mg/2 mL. The nurse would give _____ mL.

15. Zantac 15 mg, IM, q6h is prescribed. Zantac is available as 25 mg/mL. The nurse would give _____ mL.

16. Fentanyl 0.1 mg was prescribed, to be given IM, preoperatively. Fentanyl is available as 50 mcg/mL. The nurse would give _____ mL.

17. Vitamin B_{12} (cyanocobalamin) 500 mcg, IM, daily was prescribed. Vitamin B_{12} is available as 1 mg/mL. The nurse would give _____ mL.

18. The physician prescribed Apresoline 30 mg, IM, q4h. The drug is available as 20 mg/mL. The nurse would give _____ mL q4h.

19. Duralutin 375 mg, IM, q4 weeks was prescribed. The drug is available as 250 mg/mL. The nurse would give _____ mL q4 weeks.

20. The physician prescribed Primaxin 600 mg, IM, q12h. The drug is available as 750 mg/mL. The nurse would give _____ mL.

21. The physician prescribed 500 mg of Cefizox, IM, every 12 hours for a genitourinary infection. The medication is available as a powder in a 2-gram vial. Reconstitute it with 6.0 mL of sterile water for injection and shake well. Solution concentration will provide 270 mg/mL. Fluid volume will equal 7.4 mL. Use approximate quantities for dosage calculations. Give _____ mL every 12 hours.

22. Methicillin sodium 1.5 grams, IM, was prescribed for a systemic infection. Four (4) grams of the medication is available as a powder in a vial. Directions state to reconstitute it with 5.7 mL of sterile water for injection and shake well. Solution concentration will provide 500 mg/mL. To give 1.5 grams, the nurse would give _____ mL.

23. The physician prescribed 125 mg of Solu-Medrol, IM, for severe inflammation. The medication is available as a powder in a 0.5-gram vial. Reconstitute it according to directions so that each 8 mL will contain 0.5 grams of Solu-Medrol. The nurse would then give _____ mL to give 125 mg.

24. The physician prescribed 1.0 mg, IM, of leucovorin calcium, to be given once a day for the treatment of megaloblastic anemia. The medication is available as a powder in a 50-mg vial. Reconstitute it with 5.0 mL of bacteriostatic water for injection. Shake it well. Solution concentration will yield 10 mg/mL. Fluid volume will equal 5.0 mL. Give _____ mL, once a day.

25. The physician prescribed 25 mg of Librium, IM. Add 2 mL of special diluent to yield 100 mg/2 mL. The nurse should give _____ mL.

26. You are to give 20 mg of Demerol, every 6 hours postoperatively, to a 7-year-old child who weighs 20 kg. Demerol is available as 25 mg/mL. You would give _____ mL q6h.

27. The physician prescribed 5 mg of Garamycin for a child. The medication is available as 20 mg/2 mL. To give 5 mg, you would give _____ mL.

Intravenous Therapies

Intravenous fluid therapy involves the administration of water, nutrients (dextrose, protein, fats, and vitamins), electrolytes (eg, sodium, potassium, chloride), blood products, and medications. Intravenous therapies are used in patients who need fluid replacement to treat disorders like dehydration, malnutrition, electrolyte imbalance, or tissue toxicity.

Intravenous hyperalimentation (total parenteral nutrition) is used for patients who cannot ingest food orally and are in a state of *negative nitrogen balance*. Intravenous hyperalimentation provides 1.0 to 1.5 gm of protein/kg of body weight. It is administered through a large blood vessel (eg, subclavian vein). Partial parenteral nutrition, administered through a peripheral vein, is used when the dextrose concentration is <10% and therapy is < 2 weeks. Fat emulsions (eg, Intralipid) provide a concentrated form of nonprotein kilocalories (primarily unsaturated fatty acids), yielding about 1.1 kcal/mL. Fat emulsions should never be mixed with a dextrose-amino acid solution (fat emulsions will break down). A list of commonly prescribed intravenous fluids can be found in Table 13-1.

TABLE 13-1
Commonly Prescribed Intravenous Fluids

FLUIDS	ABBREVIATIONS
0.9% Sodium chloride solution	NSS
0.45% Sodium chloride solution	1/2 NSS
0.25% Sodium chloride solution	1/4 NSS
5% Dextrose in water	5% D/W D5W
10% Dextrose in water	10% D/W D10W
5% Dextrose in 0.45% sodium chloride solution	D5 1/2
Dextrose with Ringer's lactate solution	D/RL
Ringer's solution	R
Lactated Ringer's solution	RL

Plasma volume expanders
  Dextran
  Albumin	

Hyperalimentation
  Total parenteral nutrition
  Partial parenteral nutrition
	
	TPN
	PPN

Fat Emulsions Intralipid	

A physician's order for intravenous fluid therapy *must include* the type of solution, the quantity of solution, the time period for administration, and in some institutions or areas (pediatrics), the milliliters per hour. Several sample physician requests for intravenous therapy are:

+ Administer 1000 mL of D5W at 125 mL/h.
+ Administer 1000 mL of 0.9% NSS every 12 hours for 2 days.
+ Administer 500 mL of D10W at 83 mL/h.
+ Administer 100 mL of RL over 4 hours at 25 mL/h.

The physician's order is usually written as mL/h to be infused (flow rate). The flow rate is regulated either manually by straight gravity or via an electronic infusion pump or controller.

A *controller* electronically regulates drop rate by gravity, whereas an *infusion pump* consistently exerts pressure against the tubing or the fluid at a preselected rate. Both devices improve the accuracy of therapy; however, pumps can be dangerous because they continue to infuse even in the presence of infiltration or phlebitis.

There is a drip chamber at one end of the IV tubing that connects the tubing to the IV solution (bag or bottle) (see Figure 13-1). The IV solution must pass through this drip chamber, which has an opening that regulates the gtt/mL that enter the tubing. The gtt/mL (drop factor), which varies according to the manufacturer of the tubing, will be displayed on the tubing package (see Table 13-2).

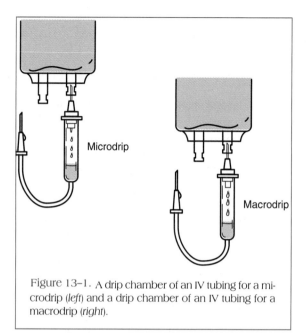

Figure 13-1. A drip chamber of an IV tubing for a microdrip (*left*) and a drip chamber of an IV tubing for a macrodrip (*right*).

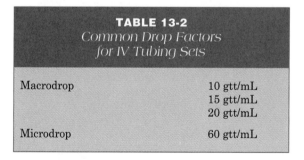

TABLE 13-2 Common Drop Factors for IV Tubing Sets	
Macrodrop	10 gtt/mL
	15 gtt/mL
	20 gtt/mL
Microdrop	60 gtt/mL

⊕ CALCULATIONS FOR REGULATING FLOW RATE

The nurse is responsible for regulating flow rate by:

- Calculating milliliters per hour (mL/h)
- Checking for the drop factor of the IV tubing
- Calculating the drops per minute (gtt/min) that are needed to deliver mL/h
- Regulating the number of drops entering the drip chamber by using the roller clamp on the tubing to adjust the flow rate (count number of drops for 1 minute)

⊕ CALCULATING MILLILITERS PER HOUR USING AN ELECTRONIC PUMP

To calculate mL/h, all you need to know is the total volume to be infused over time. When a pump or controller is used, simply set the infusion rate at the mL/h.

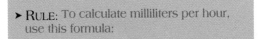

> ► RULE: To calculate milliliters per hour, use this formula:

$$\frac{\text{total volume to infuse (mL)}}{\text{total time (hours)}} = \text{milliliters per hour}$$

EXAMPLE: A patient is to receive 1000 mL of lactated Ringer's solution over a 6-hour period. The patient would receive _____ mL/hour.

Use: $$\frac{\text{total volume (mL)}}{\text{total time (hours)}}$$

= milliliters per hour

$$\frac{1000}{6} \text{ mL} = 166.6 \text{ mL/h}$$

Round off to 167 mL/h

Answer = 167 mL/h
Set infusion rate at 167 mL/H

Piggyback Delivery System. Sometimes a patient needs to receive medication in a small amount of IV solution (50–100 mL) given over a short amount of time (30 minutes). The secondary IV solution is "piggybacked" into the main IV (hung higher) or hung at the same height as the primary IV. Frequently these infusion orders do not include flow rates. To give an intermittent infusion, you will need to calculate mL/h or gtt/min (pump or controller) or gtt/min for manual management.

CALCULATING MILLILITERS PER HOUR USING AN ELECTRONIC PUMP FOR *PIGGYBACK MEDICATION*

When infusion time is less than 1 hour, use ratios and proportions and solve for *x*, mL/h. Electronic pump infusion rates are set at mL/h.

> ➤ RULE: To calculate milliliters per hour, when total time is less than 1 hour, use this formula:

$$\frac{\text{total volume}}{\text{total time (min)}} = \frac{x \,(\text{mL/h})}{60 \text{ mins}}$$

EXAMPLE: A patient is to receive 1 gram of Staphcillin in 50 mL of NSS over 30 minutes.

Use:

$$\frac{\text{total volume}}{\text{total time (min)}} = \frac{x \,(\text{mL/h})}{60 \text{ mins}}$$

$$\frac{50 \text{ mL}}{30 \text{ min}} = \frac{x \text{ mL}}{60 \text{ min}}$$

$$30x = 3000$$

$$x = \frac{3000}{30}$$

$$x = 100 \text{ mL/h}$$

Answer = Set electronic pump at 100 mL/h

CALCULATING DROPS PER MINUTE FOR GRAVITY FLOW FOR IV INFUSIONS AND PIGGYBACK MEDICATIONS

To calculate drops per minute, you need three pieces of information:

- The total volume to be infused in mL

- The drop factor of the tubing you will use
- The total time for the infusion, *in minutes*

You can use one of two methods to calculate the flow rate in drops per minute: a standard formula and a quick formula. The quick formula can be used when milliliters per hour (mL/h) replace total volume.

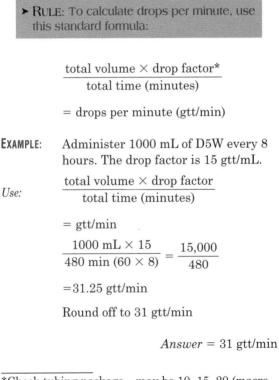

> ► RULE: To calculate drops per minute, use this standard formula:

$$\frac{\text{total volume} \times \text{drop factor*}}{\text{total time (minutes)}}$$

$$= \text{drops per minute (gtt/min)}$$

EXAMPLE: Administer 1000 mL of D5W every 8 hours. The drop factor is 15 gtt/mL.

Use: $$\frac{\text{total volume} \times \text{drop factor}}{\text{total time (minutes)}}$$

$$= \text{gtt/min}$$

$$\frac{1000 \text{ mL} \times 15}{480 \text{ min} (60 \times 8)} = \frac{15,000}{480}$$

$$= 31.25 \text{ gtt/min}$$

Round off to 31 gtt/min

Answer = 31 gtt/min

---

*Check tubing package—may be 10, 15, 20 (macro-drip) or 60 (microdrip) gtt/mL.

EXAMPLE: Administer 500 mL of 0.9% NSS over
               6 hours. The drop factor is 20 gtt/mL.

Use: $$\frac{\text{total volume} \times \text{drop factor}}{\text{total time (minutes)}}$$

               $= \text{gtt/min}$

               $$\frac{500 \text{ mL} \times 20}{360 \text{ min}} = \frac{10,000}{360}$$

               $= 27.7 \text{ gtt/min}$

               Round off to 28 gtt/min

                                       Answer $= 28 \text{ gtt/min}$

EXAMPLE: Administer 500 mL of a 5% solution
               of normal serum albumin over 30
               minutes. The drop factor is 10. Calcu-
               late the flow rate in gtt/min.

Use: $$\frac{\text{total volume} \times \text{drop factor}}{\text{total time (minutes)}}$$

               $= \text{gtt/min}$

               $$\frac{500 \text{ mL} \times 10 \text{ gtt/mL}}{30 \text{ min}} = \frac{5000}{30}$$

               $= 166 \text{ gtt/min}$

                                       Answer $= 166 \text{ gtt/min}$

EXAMPLE: Administer 500 mg of Unipen in 50 mL of D5W over 30 minutes to piggyback into main IV. Drop factor is 15 gtt/mL.

Use: $$\frac{\text{total volume} \times \text{drop factor}}{\text{total time (minutes)}} = \text{gtt/min}$$

$$\frac{50 \text{ mL} \times 15}{30} = \frac{750}{30}$$

$$= 25 \text{ gtt/min}$$

Answer = 25 gtt/min

Infusion Volume Control Sets (Buretrol, Metriset). Volume-controlled administration is used to give a small amount of solution (50–150 mL) when fluid volume needs to be carefully monitored. Medications are added into the fluid chamber through a medication port. The drop factor is always 60 gtt/mL, and the flow rate is adjusted by using a roller clamp. You must calculate gtt/min, being careful to include in the total volume any fluid used for dilution of medications.

▶ RULE: To calculate drops per minute, use this quick formula:

$$\frac{\text{milliliters per hour (mL/h)} \times \text{drop factor}}{\text{time (60 min)}}$$

$$= \text{gtt/min}$$

Using this formula requires that you know the volume (mL/h), drop factor, and time in minutes. Frequently, the physician order indicates total volume, not mL/h.

Therefore, you need to use the following to get mL/h:

$$\frac{\text{total volume (mL)}}{\text{total time (hours)}} = \text{mL/h}$$

EXAMPLE: Give 1000 mL of a drug over 10 hours. The drop factor is 20.

Calculate $\dfrac{\text{total volume (mL)}}{\text{total time (hours)}} = \text{mL/h}$
mL/h:

$$\frac{1000 \text{ mL}}{10} = 100 \text{ mL/h}$$

Use Quick $\dfrac{\text{mL/h} \times \text{drop factor}}{\text{time (60 minutes)}} = \text{gtt/min}$
Formula:

$$\frac{100 \text{ mL/h} \times 20}{60 \text{ min}} = \frac{2000}{60}$$

$$= 33.33 \text{ gtt/min}$$

Round off to 33 gtt/min

Answer = 33 gtt/min

EXAMPLE: Administer 250 mL of 0.45% NSS over 5 hours. The drop factor is 60 gtt/mL.

Calculate mL/h:	$\dfrac{\text{total volume (mL)}}{\text{total time (hours)}} = \text{mL/h}$

$$\frac{250 \text{ mL}}{5 \text{ hours}} = 50 \text{ mL/h}$$

Use Quick Formula:	$\dfrac{\text{mL/h} \times \text{drop factor}}{\text{time (60 min)}} = \text{gtt/min}$

$$\frac{50 \text{ mL/h} \times 60 \text{ gtt/mL*}}{60 \text{ min}} = \frac{3000}{60}$$

$$= 50 \text{ gtt/min}$$

Answer = 50 gtt/min

⊕ CONSTANT FACTORS

The constant factor is derived from the drop factor (of the administration set) divided into the fixed time factor of 60 minutes. It cannot be used except for time factors of 60 minutes. Because the drop factor of 60 is the same as 60 minutes, these numbers cancel themselves out. A constant factor of 1 can be used in the division to replace both of these numbers. Therefore, for this quick formula, you can use the constant factor (1) to replace 60 minutes and 60 gtt/mL.

---

*Please note: When a microdrip is used with a drop factor of 60, the gtt/min will always equal the mL/h. If the physician orders an IV to run at 75 mL/h with a microdrip, then the gtt/min is 75; if 35 mL/h, then the gtt/min is 35.

Because 60 remains constant for this quick formula, you can calculate constant factors for other drop factors by dividing by 60. Therefore, when working with a drop factor of 10, you can use the constant factor of 6 (60 ÷ 10); 15 would equal a constant factor of 4 (60 ÷ 15), and 20 would equal a constant factor of 3 (60 ÷ 20).

> ► RULE: To calculate drops per minute, use this quick formula with a constant factor:

$$\frac{\text{milliliters per hour (mL/h)}}{\text{constant factor}} = \text{gtt/min}$$

EXAMPLE: Administer 1000 mL of RL over 10 hours. The drop factor is 15 gtt/mL.

Calculate $\dfrac{\text{total volume}}{\text{total hours}} = \text{milliliters per hour}$
mL/h:

$$\frac{1000 \text{ mL}}{10 \text{ hours}} = 100 \text{ mL/h}$$

Use: $\dfrac{\text{mL/h}}{\text{constant factor}} = \text{gtt/min}$

$$\frac{100 \text{ mL/h}}{4 \ (60 \div 15)} = 25 \text{ gtt/min}$$

Answer = 25 gtt/min

► PRACTICE PROBLEMS ►

1. The physician prescribed 1000 mL of RL to infuse over 12 hours. You would give _____ mL/h.

2. You are to give 500 mL of NSS over 4 hours. You would give _____ mL/hr.

3. Administer 800 mL of NSS over 10 hours. The drop factor is 20 gtt/mL. You would give _____ gtt/min.

4. You are to give 1000 mL of 0.45% NSS to infuse over 6 hours. The drop factor is 15 gtt/mL. You would give _____ gtt/min.

5. Administer 500 mL of solution over 24 hours. The drop factor is 60 gtt/mL. You would give _____ gtt/min.

6. You are to give 600 mL of solution over 12 hours. The drop factor is 20 gtt/mL. You would give _____ gtt/min.

7. The physician prescribed an IV of 100 mL of D5W to run at 100 mL/h. The drop factor is 10. You would set the flow rate at _____ gtt/min.

8. The physician prescribed an IV of Ringer's lactate at 75 mL/h. The drop factor is 15. You would administer _____ gtt/min.

9. The physician prescribed an IV of NSS to be run at 60 mL/h. The drop factor is 20. You would run the IV at _____ gtt/min.

10. Give 1 gram of streptomycin sulfate in 75 mL of D5W over 30 minutes. The drop factor is 15 drops = 1 mL. You would piggyback this medication into the main IV and set the drop rate at _____ gtt/min.

11. The physician prescribed an IV of 1500 mL of Ringer's lactate solution to infuse over 20 hours. The drop factor is 15 gtt/mL. You would give _____ gtt/min.

12. Administer Ancef 1 gram in 50 mL of D5W over 30 minutes. The drop factor is 10 gtt/mL. The nurse would give _____ gtt/min.

13. The physician prescribed an IV of 250 mL of D5 0.22% NSS to infuse over 10 hours. The drop factor is 60 gtt/min. The nurse would give _____ mL/hr and _____ gtt/min.

14. Administer Claforan 1 gram in 100 mL of D5W to run over 30 minutes. The drop factor is 20 gtt/mL. You would give _____ gtt/min.

✚ CALCULATING INFUSION TIME

Sometimes the nurse will need to calculate the infusion time of an IV when milliliters and total volume are known. There is an easy formula to use:

> ► RULE: To calculate infusion time (total hours), use this simple formula:

$$\frac{\text{total volume}}{\text{mL/h}} = \text{infusion time (h)}$$

EXAMPLE: The physician requested that a patient receive 500 mL 0.45% NSS to infuse at 25 mL/h. Calculate the total infusion time.

Use: $$\frac{\text{total volume}}{\text{mL/h}} = \text{infusion time (h)}$$

$$\frac{500 \text{ mL}}{25 \text{ mL/h}} = 500 \div 25 = 20 \text{ hours}$$

$$Answer = 20 \text{ hours}$$

Occasionally, you will need to determine infusion time when mL/h is not provided. Follow this rule:

> ► RULE: To calculate infusion time, use this simple formula when mL/h is unknown:

- Convert gtt/min to mL/min.
- Convert mL/min to mL/h.
- Use the following formula:

$$\frac{\text{total volume}}{\text{mL/h}} = \text{infusion time (h)}$$

EXAMPLE: The physician prescribed 1000 mL of RL to run at 30 gtt/min, using a drop factor of 15 gtt/mL.

Convert   15 gtt : 1 mL :: 30 gtt : x mL
gtt/min to
mL/min:

$$15 \times x = 1 \times 30$$
$$15x = 30$$
$$x = 2 \text{ mL/min}$$

Convert   2 mL/min $\times$ 60 min = 120 mL/h
mL/min to
mL/h:

Use: $\dfrac{\text{total volume}}{\text{mL/h}}$ = infusion time

$\dfrac{1000 \text{ mL}}{120 \text{ mL/h}}$ = 1000 ÷ 120 = 8.3 hours

Convert: (0.3 h = $\dfrac{3}{10} \times 60$ min = 18 min)

Answer = 8 hours and 18 min

✦ SPECIAL CONSIDERATIONS

INTERMITTENT INTRAVENOUS INFUSION

Heparin Lock. A heparin lock has a needle or catheter that is attached to a short tubing with an injection port on the end. It provides for intermittent IV infusion; therefore, the patient's mobility is not restricted by an IV that is in place but only used intermittently for infusions.

PEDIATRIC INTRAVENOUS MEDICATIONS

It is essential that pediatric intravenous therapy be as exact as possible because infants and children have a narrow range of fluid balance. Therefore, a volume-controlled infusion set is recommended, and total fluid volume consists of medication diluent volume, IV solution volume, and flush volume (5–15 mL). An electronic pump or controller is almost always used to regulate the infusion.

CALCULATING PEDIATRIC FLOW RATE

> ► RULE: To calculate flow rate (drops per minute), use the standard or quick formula. Total volume must include IV solution volume, medication dilution volume, and flush volume.

EXAMPLE: Give 250 mg of an antibiotic in 20 mL of D5 0.45% NSS to infuse over 30 minutes. Follow with a 10-mL flush. The drop factor is 60 gtt/mL.

Use: $$\frac{\text{total volume} \times \text{drop factor}}{\text{total time (minutes)}}$$

$$= \text{gtt/min}$$

$$\frac{20 \text{ mL of solution} + 10 \text{ mL of flush} \times 60 \text{ gtt/mL}}{30 \text{ minutes}}$$

$$= \frac{1800}{30} = 60 \text{ gtt/min}$$

Determine   The antibiotic requires 5 mL for
Reconstituted   drug reconstitution.
Drug Volume:

Fill Chamber: Run in 15 mL of IV solution (20
                  mL–5 mL needed for drug
                  dilution). Add remaining 5 mL with
                  reconstituted drug.

Set Rate: Set rate at 60 gtt/min.

Add Flush: When medication is absorbed, add
                  10 mL of flush and keep flow rate
                  at 60 gtt/min.

CRITICAL CARE APPLICATIONS

In critical care situations, physicians order IV
medications by flow rate (gtt/mL/h) or by drug
dosage (mg/min or mg/h, mcg/kg/min). You must
always calculate a safe dosage range before you
give the IV.

CALCULATING DRUG DOSAGE PER HOUR OR PER MINUTE.

> ► RULE: To calculate drug dosage per hour
>   or per minute, follow these steps:

- ◆ Determine mg/h if you have mL/h by using
  ratios and proportions.
- ◆ Convert mg/h to mg/min and/or mcg/min.

EXAMPLE: Give dopamine HCl 600 mg in 500
                mL D5W at 20 mL/h. Calculate the
                dosage in mcg/min. Is this safe for a
                patient who weighs 100 kg?

Complete the Proportion: 600 mg : 500 mL :: x mg : 20 mL

$500 \times x = 600 \times 20$

$500\, x = 12{,}000$

$\dfrac{500x}{500} = \dfrac{12{,}000}{500}$

$x = \dfrac{12{,}000}{500}$

Reduce: $\dfrac{12{,}000}{500} = 24$ mg/h

Convert mg to mcg: 24 mg $\times$ 1000 = 24,000 mcg/h

Change mcg/h to mcg/min: 24,000 mcg/h $\div$ 60 min = 400 mcg/min

Determine safe dosage range: Safe dosage for dopamine HCl IV is 2–5 mcg/kg/min. The safe dosage range for 100 kg is 200 mcg/min to 500 mcg/min.

Answer = 400 mcg/min; dosage is within safe range

⊕ CALCULATING MILLILITERS PER HOUR

> ► RULE: To calculate mL/h for drugs ordered in mg/min, follow these steps:

♦ Calculate mL/min using the following formula:

$$\frac{D}{H} \times Q = x$$

- Calculate mL/h by multiplying mL/min $\times$ 60 min.
- Estimate gtt/min, if necessary, using the quick formula (refer to page 183–184 to review).

EXAMPLE: The physician prescribed lidocaine 1 gram in 500 mL D5W to infuse at 2 mg/min. Determine flow rate.

Use: $\qquad \frac{D}{H} \times Q = x$

$$\frac{2 \text{ mg/min}}{1 \text{ g (1000 mg)}} \times 500 \text{ mL} = x$$

$$\frac{2 \times 500}{1000} = \frac{1000}{1000} = 1 \text{ mL/min}$$

Calculate $\quad$ 1 mL/min $\times$ 60 min = 60 mL/h
mL/h:

$$Answer = 60 \text{ mL/h}$$

END OF CHAPTER REVIEW

Complete the following IV calculations:

1. To infuse 500 mL of solution over 8 hours, you would give _____ mL/h.

2. Administer 1000 mL over 10 hours. You would give _____ mL/h.

3. To deliver 1000 mL of D5 0.45% NSS over 4 hours, the nurse would have to administer _____ mL/h.

4. To deliver 500 mL of D5W over a 6-hour period, the nurse would set the flow rate to deliver _____ mL/h.

5. To deliver 250 mL of NSS over a 5-hour period, the nurse would set the flow rate to deliver _____ mL/h.

6. A patient is to receive 500 mL of 0.45% NSS with 20 mEq of KCl to run over 8 hours. The drop factor is 20 gtt/mL. The nurse would give _____ mL/h.

7. Administer 1000 mL of 0.9% NSS over 8 hours. The drop factor is 10 gtt/mL. The flow rate would be _____ gtt/min.

8. Administer 500 mL of D5W over a 12-hour period as KVO. The microdrip provides 60 gtt/mL. Use the Quick Formula with a constant factor. The flow rate would be _____ gtt/min.

9. To administer 1.0 liter of Ringer's lactate over 6 hours, you would give _____ mL/h. The drop factor is 10 gtt/mL. The flow rate would be _____ gtt/min.

10. The physician prescribed 1000 mL of D5W to infuse over 24 hours. With a drop factor of 15 gtt/mL, you would give _____ gtt/min. Use the Quick Formula with a constant factor.

11. The physician prescribed 1000 mL of D5W 0.9% NSS to infuse at 75 mL/h. The drop factor is 15 gtt/mL. You would give _____ gtt/min.

12. Ringer's lactate, 500 mL, is to infuse at 50 mL/h. The drop factor is 10. You would set the rate at _____ gtt/min. Use the Quick Formula with a constant factor.

13. Administer 1000 mL of RL at 50 mL/h. The
    total infusion time would be _____ hours.

14. You are to give 500 mL of NSS at 40 mL/h.
    The total infusion time would be _____ hours.

15. The physician prescribed 250 mL of D5W at
    20 mL/h. The total infusion time would be
    _____ hours.

16. The physician prescribed 100 mL of albumin
    to be absorbed over 2 hours. The drop factor
    is 15 gtt/mL. The nurse would run the IV at
    _____ gtt/min.

17. A patient is to receive 1000 mL of NSS with
    20,000 units of heparin over 24 hours. The
    drop factor is 60 gtt/mL. The nurse would
    give _____ gtt/min.

18. A patient is to receive 350 mg of aminoph-
    ylline in 150 mL of D5W over a 1-hour
    period of time. The drop factor is 15 gtt/mL.
    The nurse would give _____ gtt/min.

19. Administer 100 mL of an antibiotic solution
    via a volume control set over 60 minutes.
    The microdrip provides 60 gtt/mL. You would
    give _____ gtt/min.

20. A child is to receive 30 mL of an intravenous
    solution every hour through a volume
    control set that delivers 60 minidrops/mL.
    The flow rate should be set at _____ gtt/min
    to deliver 30 mL/hour.

21. Give a child aminophylline 250 mg IVPB in 50 mL of NSS over 1 hour via a Buretrol. Aminophylline is available in 250 mg/10 mL. Follow with 10 mL of flush. You would give _____ gtt/min with a total volume of _____ mL.

22. A hypertensive patient weighs 165 pounds. His physician prescribed Nipride 3 mcg/kg/minute, IV. To administer, 50 mg of Nipride has to be added to a 250-mL solution of D5W. This solution would contain a concentration of Nipride, _____ mcg/mL. Using an infusion pump, the nurse would set the flow rate at _____ mL/h.

23. The physician prescribed Mithracin 25 mcg/kg by slow IV infusion for a patient who weighs 154 pounds. Mithracin is available in a vial labeled 2.5 mg/mL. To prepare the correct dose, the nurse would add _____ mL of Mithracin to 1000 mL of D5W.

24. A patient is to receive Nitrostat 20 mcg/min, IV. Nitrostat is available in a 10-mL vial labeled 5 mg/mL. To prepare a 40-mcg/mL solution, the nurse would add _____ mL of Nitrostat to a 250-mL D5W IV bottle and set the infusion pump flow rate at _____ mL/h to deliver 20 mcg/min.

25. The physician prescribed 500 mL of a 10% Intralipid solution to infuse over 4 hours. Using a controller, the nurse would set the rate at _____ mL/h.

26. The patient is to receive 150 mg of Dilantin by slow IV push for status epilepticus. Dilantin is labeled 50 mg/mL. The nurse would give _____ mL over a 10-minute period.

27. Give 500 mg of dopamine in 500 mL of D5 NSS to infuse at 300 mcg/min. Calculate flow rate in mL/h. You would give _____ mL/h to deliver _____ mg/h.

28. The physician prescribed morphine sulfate 1 gram in 100 mL D5 NSS to infuse at 10 mg per hour. Calculate the flow rate in gtt/min. You would give _____ gtt/min using a microdrip.

29. The physician prescribed Solu-Medrol 20 mg by slow IV push for an asthmatic child. Solu-Medrol is labeled 40 mg/mL. The nurse would give _____ mL over 3 minutes.

30 An infant is to receive 15 mL of D5 0.22% NSS solution every hour through a volume control set that delivers 60 microdrops/mL. The flow rate should be set at _____ gtt/min to deliver 15 mL/hr.

31. A child is to receive ampicillin 250 mg IVPB in 25 mL of NSS over 1 hour via a Buretrol. Ampicillin 500 mg/10 mL is available. Follow with 10 mL of flush. The nurse would give _____ gtt/min with the total volume of _____ mL.

32. A patient is to receive 1200 mL of RL to run over 12 hours. The drop factor is 20 gtt/mL. The nurse would give _____ mL/hr and _____ gtt/min.

14

Drugs Measured in USP Units

Drugs are measured in units when strength can be more accurately determined than weight. There are three major drugs that are measured in units: heparin, penicillin, and insulin; however, a unit of insulin is not considered the same as a unit of heparin or penicillin. Dosage calculations for heparin and penicillin are solved using this formula: D/H $\times$ Q = amount to give.

INSULIN

Insulin is a natural hormone secreted by the Islets of Langerhans in the pancreas to maintain blood sugar. It is easy to prepare insulin for injection. Insulin is most commonly packaged in vials of 100 units/mL (U = 100/mL), and the standard insulin syringe is calibrated in 100 units/mL. Medication orders are written in units/mL.

The most common U-100 syringe is calibrated every 2 units, with every 10th unit marked in large numbers on one side (Figure 14-1A). A double scale U-100 syringe has 2-unit calibrations. Every 5 units is marked in large numbers on the left side, and every 10 units is marked on the right side. This makes it easier to accurately measure odd and even unit increments.

A Lo-Dose® insulin syringe is calibrated every unit for 50 U/0.5 mL; every 5 units are marked (Figure 14-1B). Pediatric doses can be given in a 30-U/0.5-mL syringe (Figure 14-1C). The enlarged scale of the Lo-Dose® syringe makes it easier to read.

Insulin orders are written in units/mL, and U-100 strength is used almost exclusively. With

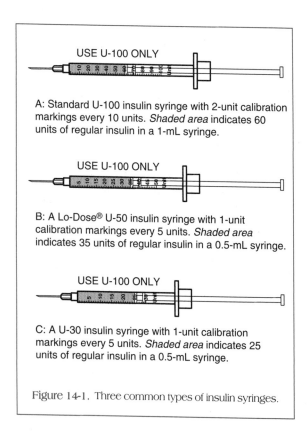

USE U-100 ONLY

A: Standard U-100 insulin syringe with 2-unit calibration markings every 10 units. *Shaded area* indicates 60 units of regular insulin in a 1-mL syringe.

USE U-100 ONLY

B: A Lo-Dose® U-50 insulin syringe with 1-unit calibration markings every 5 units. *Shaded area* indicates 35 units of regular insulin in a 0.5-mL syringe.

USE U-100 ONLY

C: A U-30 insulin syringe with 1-unit calibration markings every 5 units. *Shaded area* indicates 25 units of regular insulin in a 0.5-mL syringe.

Figure 14-1. Three common types of insulin syringes.

U-100 medication orders, all you have to do is draw up the desired dose by filling the insulin syringe to the identified calibration. Mathematical calculations are not required.

> ➤ RULE: To prepare insulin for injection, follow these steps:

- Read the medication order, noting the type of insulin and unit preparation desired. For example, a patient is ordered 60 units of NPH insulin.
- Select the insulin. Check the label three times. You would choose the vial of NPH insulin marked 100 units/mL.
- Match the insulin syringe to the unit preparation of insulin. You should choose a U-100 syringe because the insulin preparation comes in a vial marked 100 U/mL.
- Draw up the required dose by filling the syringe to the desired calibration. You would fill a U-100 syringe to the 60 units calibration.

MIXING TWO TYPES OF INSULIN

Frequently you will find it necessary to mix two types of insulin, usually regular and NPH. When you have to mix insulins, there are five important guidelines that you must remember:

1. Do not contaminate the contents of one vial with the contents of the other vial.
2. Always draw up *regular insulin first.*
3. Always *draw up the NPH insulin last* because chemically it has a protein substance in it that regular insulin does not have. Drawing up the NPH insulin last helps prevent contamination of the regular insulin.
4. Choose a Lo-Dose® insulin syringe (U-30 or U-50) to measure low dosages; use a U-100 syringe for insulin combinations > 50 U.
5. Always add air into each vial equal to the amount of the required dose. Air prevents a vacuum from occurring. ***Note:*** Always inject air into the *NPH vial first!*

> ▶ RULE: To mix two types of insulin in one syringe for injection, regular and NPH, follow these steps:

- Check the medication order. Know the total number of units needed.
- Wash your hands and obtain the correct vials of insulin and the correct syringes. Both should be in the same unit of strength (U-100).
- Wipe the top of both vials with an alcohol swab. Regular is always clear and colorless in appearance. NPH is cloudy in appearance. Rotate the vial of NPH between your palms.
- Inject air equal to the insulin dose of NPH (10 units) into the NPH insulin vial first (**A** on p. 201). *Do not touch the insulin with the needle.* Withdraw the needle.

- Use the same syringe and inject air equal to the dose of regular insulin (30 units) into the regular insulin vial **(B)**. Be careful that the needle does not touch the solution because air should not be bubbled through the solution.
- Invert the vial of regular insulin and draw back the required dosage **(C)**. Check the dosage (30 units).
- Remove the needle from the vial of regular insulin **(D)** and check for air bubbles. Tap the syringe to remove any bubbles. If necessary, draw up additional medication for correct dosage.

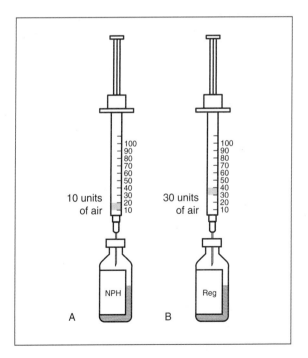

- Put the needle into the NPH vial **(E)**, being careful not to inject any regular insulin into the NPH vial.
- Invert the vial of NPH and withdraw the required dosage (10 units) while holding the syringe at eye level. There should be a total of 40 units **(F)**.
- Check the dosage, which should be the addition of the two insulin orders **(G)**. Air bubbles at this point indicate an incorrect dose, and the medication must be drawn up again.
- Prepare to administer the correct dose.

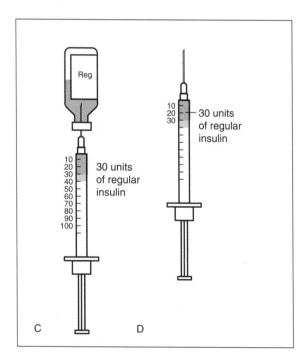

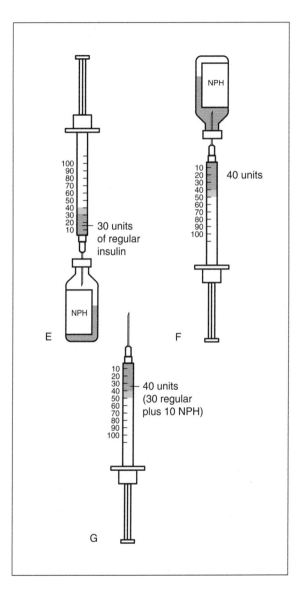

30 units of regular insulin

40 units

40 units (30 regular plus 10 NPH)

E

F

G

➤ PRACTICE PROBLEMS ➤

Look at the following syringes and identify the correct dosage by using an arrow to mark your answer or shade in the areas.

1. Indicate 60 units U-100 insulin.

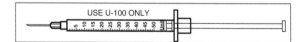

2. Indicate 82 units U-100 insulin.

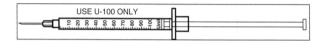

3. Indicate 45 units U-100 insulin.

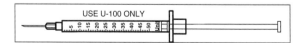

4. Indicate 35 units U-100 insulin.

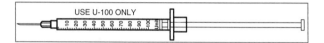

5. Indicate 10 units regular U-100 insulin combined with 16 units of NPH U-100 insulin.

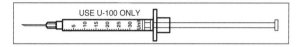

6. Indicate 16 units of Lente U-100 insulin combined with 40 units of NPH U-100 insulin.

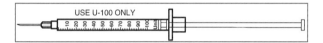

Identify the insulin dosage indicated by the shaded area on the following syringes.

7.

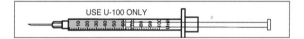

_____units

8.

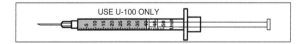

_____units

9.

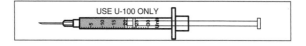

_____units

10.

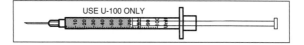

_____units

For the combined doses of insulin, indicate the total insulin dosage in the first column and the appropriate syringe (U-30, U-50, or U-100) in the second column.

	Total Dosage	Syringe/mL
11. 5 U regular 16 U NPH	_____	_____
12. 15 U Ultralente 30 U regular	_____	_____
13. 28 U regular 36 U Lente	_____	_____
14. 18 U regular 20 U NPH	_____	_____
15. 20 U Lente 36 U regular	_____	_____

⊕ INSULIN DELIVERY SYSTEMS

Insulin is also available for injection in 1.5-mL cartridges (100 units/mL [U-100]) for use with NovoPen® and Novolin Pen® insulin delivery systems (see Figure 14-2). The cartridges deliver 2–36 units of insulin in 2-unit increments by a push of the plunger mechanism. The insulin delivery devices look like a fountain pen, are about 6 inches long, weigh 5 to 7 ounces, and are designed for patients to give themselves insulin by using a push-button/plunger mechanism. Both systems use PenNeedle® disposable needles and Novolin® insulin: regular, NPH, or a combination of NPH (70%) and regular (30%). Medication orders are written in insulin units. Mathematical calculations are not required. Your responsibilities include assessing the patient's ability to assemble the equipment, helping the patient with it as necessary, checking the accuracy of the dose delivered, evaluating the patient's response to the medication, and documenting that the dosage was given as prescribed. You should refer to product literature (available from Novo Nordisk*) for specific instructions on assembly and injection.

---

*Novo Nordisk, 100 Overlook Center, Princeton, NJ 08540-7810, (609) 987-5800.

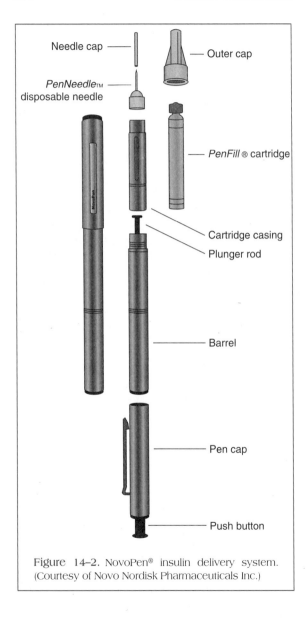

Figure 14-2. NovoPen® insulin delivery system. (Courtesy of Novo Nordisk Pharmaceuticals Inc.)

⊕ HEPARIN

CALCULATING HEPARIN FOR SUBCUTANEOUS INJECTION

Heparin is an anticoagulant that is ordered SC or IV (for intermittent or continuous infusion). To safely administer heparin, you must first determine that the prescribed dose is within normal limits. Then you need to calculate, for IV infusion, units per hour or milliliters per hour using the ratio-proportion method.

> ➤ RULE: The normal heparinizing adult dosage is 20,000 U to 40,000 U/24 hours.

* To calculate the 24-hour dosage, simply estimate the 24-hour total.

CALCULATE HEPARIN FOR SUBCUTANEOUS INJECTION

> ➤ RULE: To prepare heparin for subcutaneous injection, follow these steps:

* Read the medication order, noting the number of units to be administered. For example, a patient is prescribed 3000 units of heparin to be administered subcutaneously every 12 hours.

- Determine if the prescribed dose is within the normal heparinizing adult dosage for 24 hours. Heparin 3000 U q12h = 6000 U/24 hours. This is below the normal dosage range and is safe to give.
- Select the appropriate ampule/vial. For example, you choose a 10-mL multidose vial in a concentration of 5000 units/mL.
- Choose a 1.0-mL syringe.

Use: $\dfrac{D}{H} \times Q = x$

$$\frac{3000 \text{ U}}{5000 \text{ U}} = \frac{3}{5}$$

$$\frac{3}{5} \times 1.0 \text{ mL (quantity)} = 0.6 \text{ mL}$$

Answer = 0.6 mL

CALCULATING HEPARIN FOR INTRAVENOUS INFUSION

> ▶ RULE: To calculate hourly dosage of heparin for intravenous infusion, follow these steps:

- Use ratios and proportions to determine the hourly units of heparin if the mL/h infusion is known.
- Calculate the mL/h infusion first if the drop factor (gtt/mL) and flow rate (gtt/min) are known.

- ◆ Determine if the dosage is within the normal heparinizing adult dosage (20,000–40,000 U every 24 hours) by calculating the 24-hour dosage.

EXAMPLE: Give 1000 mL of D5W with 30,000 units of heparin to infuse at 30 mL/h. Calculate the hourly dosage of heparin.

Complete the proportion to calculate units/hour:

30,000 U : 1000 mL :: xU : 30 mL

$$1000 \times x = 30{,}000 \times 30$$

$$1000x = 900{,}000$$

$$x = \frac{\cancel{900{,}000}}{\cancel{1000}_1} = 900$$

$x = 900$ U in 30 mL to infuse per hour

Answer = 900 U/h

Estimate 24-hour dosage:

900 U/h $\times$ 24 h = 21,600 U/24 h. This is within normal range for adult dosage.

EXAMPLE: Give 1000 mL D5W with 20,000 U of heparin by straight gravity flow infusion. The drop factor is 10 gtt/mL, and the IV flow rate is 10 gtt/min. Calculate the hourly dosage of heparin.

Calculate mL/min: 10 gtt : 1 mL :: 10 gtt : x mL

$$10x = 10$$

$$x = 1 \text{ mL/min}$$

Change mL/min to mL/h: 1 mL/min × 60 min = 60 mL/h

Complete the proportion to calculate units/hour: 20,000 U : 1000 mL :: xU : 60 mL

$$1000 \times x = 20,000 \times 60$$

Solve for x: $1000x = 1,200,000$

$$\frac{1000x}{1000} = \frac{1,200,000}{1000}$$

$$x = \frac{\cancel{1,200,000}^{1200}}{\cancel{1000}_1}$$

$$x = 1200 \text{ U in 60 mL to infuse per hour}$$

Estimate 24-hour dosage: 1200 U × 24 h = 28,800/24 h. This is within normal range for adult dosage.

Answer = 1200 U/h

CALCULATING HEPARIN FLOW RATE

> ➤ RULE: To calculate heparin flow rate
> when heparin is ordered in units per
> hour, follow these steps

+ Use the ratio-proportion method to calculate
  the flow rate in mL/h if the infusion is by
  pump.
+ Calculate the flow rate in gtt/min if the
  infusion is by gravity. Use the Quick
  Formula with a constant factor (review
  pages 183–184).

EXAMPLE: Give 1000 U/h of heparin IV. You have
500 mL of D5W with 20,000 U of heparin added. The drop factor is 15
gtt/mL. Calculate the flow rate.

Complete   20,000 U : 500 mL :: 1000 U : x mL
the
proportion:

$$20{,}000x = 500 \times 1000$$

Solve for x: $20{,}000x = 500{,}000$

$$\frac{20{,}000x}{20{,}000} = \frac{500{,}000}{20{,}000}$$

$$x = \frac{\overset{1}{\cancel{20{,}000}}x}{\cancel{20{,}000}_{\uparrow}} = \frac{\overset{25}{\cancel{500{,}000}}}{\cancel{20{,}000}_{\uparrow}}$$

$$x = 25 \text{ mL/h}$$

Calculate
gtt/min— $$\frac{\text{mL/h}}{\text{constant factor}} = \text{gtt/min}$$
use:

$$\frac{25 \text{ mL/h}}{4} = 6.25 \text{ gtt/min}$$

Round off to 6 gtt/min

Answer = 6 gtt/min

EXAMPLE: Give 600 U/h of heparin IV. You have
               500 mL of D5W with 25,000 U of hep-
               arin added. The drop factor is 60
               gtt/min (microdrops). Calculate the
               flow rate.

Complete   25,000 U : 500 mL :: 600 U : x mL
the
proportion:

               $25,000\, x = 500 \times 600$

Solve for x: $25,000\, x = 300,000$

$$\frac{25{,}000x}{25{,}000} = \frac{300{,}000}{25{,}000}$$

$$\frac{\cancel{25{,}000}^{1}x}{\cancel{25{,}000}_{1}} = \frac{\cancel{300{,}000}^{12}}{\cancel{25{,}000}_{1}}$$

               $x = 12$ mL/h

Calculate
gtt/min—
use:

$$\frac{mL/h}{\text{constant factor}} = gtt/min$$

$$\frac{12\ mL/h}{1} = 12\ gtt/min$$

Answer = 12 gtt/min

HEPARIN LOCK FLUSH SOLUTION

Heparin sodium lock flush solution contains a small dose of heparin and is used to maintain the patency of intravenous catheters. The hep-lock flush solution contains 10 or 100 units/milliliter. It is administered after a normal saline flush, which follows administration of an intravenous medication, usually an antibiotic. Winthrop has manufactured a Hep-Pak® convenience package for heparin lock flush procedures. The Hep-Pak® contains one cartridge of heparin lock flush solution (10–100 U/mL) and two cartridges of sodium chloride solution.

➤ PRACTICE PROBLEMS ➤

1. Give 500 mL of D5 NSS with 10,000 units of heparin to infuse at 20 mL/h. Calculate the hourly dosage of heparin. Is the dosage within the normal, safe range for 24 hours?

Answer = _____ U/h. Safe?_____

2. Give 100 mL of D5W with 20,000 U of heparin IV. The drop factor is 20 gtt/mL, and the IV flow rate is 10 gtt/min. Calculate the hourly dosage of heparin. Is the dosage within the normal, safe range for 24 hours? _____

3. Give 800 U of heparin IV every hour. You have 1000 mL of D5 NSS with 40,000 U of heparin added. The drop factor is 60 gtt/min. Calculate the flow rate.

   Answer = _____ mL/h _____gtt/min

⊕ PENICILLIN

Some preparations of penicillin come in units/mL, whereas others come in milligrams/mL. You can use ratios and proportions or the formula D/H × Q = amount to give.

> ► RULE: To prepare penicillin for injection, follow these steps:

- Read the medication order, noting the number of units to be administered. For example, a patient is prescribed 300,000 units of penicillin G procaine to be administered q12 hours.
- Penicillin G procaine is available as 600,000 units/1.2 mL. Therefore, you would use the following formula:

$$\frac{D}{H} \times Q = x$$

EXAMPLE: $\dfrac{300,000 \text{ U}}{600,000 \text{ U}} = \dfrac{3}{6} = \dfrac{1}{2}$

$\dfrac{1}{2} \times 1.2 \text{ mL} = 0.6 \text{ mL}$

Answer = 0.6 mL

END OF CHAPTER REVIEW

Complete the following problems:

1. The physician orders 30 U of U-100 NPH insulin to be given before lunch. You would select a _____ syringe and draw up _____ U of NPH.

2. You have been asked to give 15 U of Humulin R insulin and 24 U of U-100 NPH. You would give a combined dose of _____ units in a _____ syringe.

3. The physician prescribed 15 units of Humulin R insulin to be given subcutaneously at 11:00 AM to cover an "Accucheck" reading of 325. The nurse had a U-30 syringe. She would draw up into the syringe _____ units.

4. The physician prescribed 50 units of Humulin N insulin to be given subcutaneously at 8:00 AM. Using a U-100 insulin syringe, the nurse would draw up _____ units.

5. The physician prescribed a combination of
   22 units of NPH insulin and 12 units of
   regular insulin. Using a U-100 insulin
   syringe, the nurse would draw up a total of
   _____ units, making certain to draw up the
   _____ insulin last.

6. To help a patient give himself 6 units of
   Novolin® R insulin using a NovoPen®, the
   nurse would remind the patient to depress
   the push button _____ times because each
   depression releases _____ units of insulin.

7. A patient is to receive 10,000 units of heparin
   subcutaneously at 8:00 AM and 8:00 PM for 5
   days. Heparin sodium for injection is
   available in a TUBEX Cartridge-Needle unit
   in 15,000 units per mL. The nurse would give
   _____ mL every 12 hours for a daily total
   dosage of _____ U/24 hours. This is/is not
   within the normal dosage range. _____

8. Heparin sodium, 8000 units, is to be given
   subcutaneously, every 8 hours. The
   medication is available in a vial labeled
   10,000 units per milliliter. The nurse would
   give _____ mL every 8 hours for a total
   dosage of _____ U/24 h. This is/is not within
   the normal dosage range. _____

9. The physician prescribed heparin sodium,
   5000 units, subcutaneously, twice a day.
   Heparin is available in a vial labeled 7500
   units per milliliter. The nurse would give
   _____ mL twice a day for a total dosage of
   _____ U/24 h. This is/is not within the
   normal dosage range. _____

10. The physician prescribed 5000 units of heparin for injection intravenously through a heparin lock. Heparin is available in a 10-mL vial in a concentration of 20,000 units per milliliter. The nurse would administer _____ mL.

11. The physician ordered 500 mL of D5W with 30,000 units of heparin to infuse at 10 mL/h. Calculate the hourly dosage of heparin: _____ U/h in 10 mL.

12. The physician prescribed 1000 mL of 0.45% NSS with 15,000 U of heparin IV. The drop factor is 10 gtt/mL, and the IV flow rate is 15 gtt/min. Calculate the hourly dosage of heparin. _____ mL/min = _____ mL/h; give _____ U/h = _____ U/24 h.

13. You are to give 500 U of heparin IV hourly. You have 1000 mL D5W with 10,000 U of heparin added. The drop factor is 20 gtt/mL. Calculate the flow rate. _____ mL/h will be infused at _____ gtt/min.

14. The physician prescribed Crysticillin 600,000 units IM as a single dose. Crysticillin is available in a 12-mL vial labeled 500,000 units per milliliter. The nurse would give _____ mL.

15. The physician prescribed 300,000 units of Bicillin intramuscularly every 12 hours for 5 days. Bicillin is packaged as 600,000 units/mL. The nurse would give _____ mL every 12 hours.

16. The physician prescribed penicillin G
    potassium 125,000 units, IM, every 12
    hours. The medication is available in
    solution as 250,000 units/5 mL. The nurse
    would give _____ mL every 12 hours.

17. Penicillin G benzathine 1.2 million units was
    prescribed, IM, as a single injection. The
    medication is available as 300,000 units per
    milliliter. The nurse would give _____ mL.

18. A patient is to receive 500 mL of D5W with
    15,000 units of heparin over 24 hours. The
    drop factor is 60 gtt/mL. Using an infusion
    pump, the nurse would set the flow rate at
    _____ mL/h to deliver _____ units/hour of
    heparin.

19. Give 500 units/h of heparin IV. You have 500
    mL of D5W with 10,000 units of heparin
    added. The drop factor is 15 gtt/mL.
    Calculate the flow rate. _____

20. The physician prescribed 10 units of
    Humulin R insulin and 22 units of U-100
    NPH. You would give a combined dose of
    _____ units in a _____ syringe.

15

Immunostimulants: Vaccines, Toxoids, and Immune Serum Globulins

Vaccines and toxoids contain particles of bacteria or viruses that have been killed or are less virulent than the original pathogen. They provide *active immunity* by triggering an immune response that would occur if a person had become infected. Examples include DPT triple antigen, hepatitis B vaccine, rabies vaccine, and poliovirus vaccine. Research is ongoing in an effort to develop an AIDS vaccine. Immune serum globulins provide *passive immunity* by supplying antibodies from a previously infected source to a person who may be or has been exposed to an infectious agent. Examples include varicella-zoster immune globulin, hepatitis B immune globulin, and RhoGAM.

Immunostimulants are available in milliliters or international units (IUs) and are administered intradermally, subcutaneously, and intramuscularly. Rules for drug preparation can be found in Chapters 12 and 13. Appendices B, C, and D will provide a helpful review of administration techniques.

END OF CHAPTER REVIEW

Complete the following problems

1. A physician prescribed 0.5 mL of Hibivax, subcutaneously, for a 4-year-old. The nurse should reconstitute it with 6 mL of the diluent provided by the manufacturer. The vial will provide 10 doses. The nurse would give _____ mL.

2. A patient is to receive 0.5 mL of rubella virus vaccine, subcutaneously. Reconstitute it, using the entire amount of diluent supplied by the manufacturer. The nurse would give _____ mL.

3. A physician prescribes rabies immune globulin, 20 units/kg, IM, for a patient who weighs 145 pounds. The rabies immune globulin is labeled 150 units/mL. The nurse would give _____ mL.

4. A patient is to receive 500 units of tetanus immune globulin, IM. The medication is available as 250 units/mL. The nurse would give _____ mL.

5. The nurse is to administer 625 units of varicella-zoster immune globulin, IM. The medication is labeled 125 units/2.5 mL. The nurse would give _____ mL.

6. Hepatitis B immune globulin 0.06 mL/kg is prescribed IM for a patient who weighs 110 pounds. The nurse would give _____ mL.

7. The physician prescribed immune globulin 0.25 mL/kg, IM, for postexposure prophylaxis of measles. The patient weighs 119 pounds. The nurse would give _____ mL.

8. The physician prescribed 25 mg, IM, of Hib-Immune. Hib-Immune is labeled 25 mg/0.5 mL. The drug requires reconstitution with the diluent provided by the manufacturer. To give 25 mg, the nurse would give _____ mL.

9. Gammar 0.06 mL/kg was prescribed for a 132-pound female who had been exposed to hepatitis B. The nurse would give _____ mL within 1 week of exposure. (If > 3.0 mL is required, divide the dosage into two injections.)

10. The nurse is to administer 0.5 mL of DTAP vaccine, IM. The vial of DTaP is a multiple-dose vial of 10 mL. The nurse would give _____ mL. The vial contains _____ doses of DTaP.

11. The physician prescribed 25 mg of Varivax vaccine, subcutaneously. The vaccine is labeled 50 mg/mL. The nurse would give _____ mL.

16

Solutions

Solutions are mixtures of liquids, solids, or gases (known as *solutes*) that are dissolved in a diluent (known as a *solvent*). Solutions can be administered externally (compresses, soaks, baths) or internally (irrigations, lavages), and they are usually prepared by a pharmacist or packaged by a pharmaceutical company. However, the preparation of solutions may increasingly become a nurse's responsibility as nursing's role outside the hospital institution expands to the home health care arena.

Solutions can be prepared from full-strength drugs or from stock solutions. Full-strength drugs are considered to be 100% pure, whereas stock solutions contain drugs in a given solution strength, always less than 100%, from which weaker solutions are made. Solution strengths can be expressed in a percentage or ratio format.

Solution problems are basically problems involving percents that can be solved using the ratio-proportion method. When setting up the ratios and proportions for a solution made from a pure drug or from a stock solution, *use the strength of the desired solution to the strength of the available solution as one ratio, and the solute to the solution as the other ratio.* Look at the following proportion.

desired solution strength : available solution strength :: amount of solute : total amount of solution

You can substitute an abbreviated formula when using a proportion for a solution made from a stock solution:

$$\frac{\text{desired strength}}{\text{on-hand strength}} \times \text{total amount of solution}$$

$$= \text{amount of solute needed}$$

$$\left[\frac{D}{H} \times Q = x \right]$$

When calculating solution problems, it is important to remember two things:

1. Work within the same measurement system (milligrams with milliliters, grains with minims).
2. Change solutions expressed in the fraction or colon format to a percent (1:2 or 1/2 should be equal to 50%).

PREPARING A SOLUTION FROM A SOLUTION OR PURE DRUG

EXAMPLE: Prepare 500 mL of a 5% boric acid solution from pure boric acid crystals.

Proportion: $\dfrac{D}{H} \times Q = x$

$$\frac{5.0\%}{100\%} = \frac{50}{1000} = \frac{1}{20}$$

$$\frac{1}{20} \times 500 \text{ mL} = 25 \text{ g}$$

Answer = 25 grams*

Answer = 25 grams; weigh and dissolve
25 grams in 500 cc of water.

EXAMPLE: Prepare 1.0 liter of a 10% solution
from a pure drug.

Proportion: $\dfrac{D}{H} \times Q = x$

$$\frac{10\%}{100\%} = \frac{10}{100} = \frac{1}{10}$$

$$\frac{1}{10} \times 1000 \text{ mL} = 100 \text{ mL}$$

Answer = 100 mL

Answer = Measure 100 mL of pure drug
and add 900 mL of water to prepare
1.0 liter of a 10% solution.

---

*The answer is in grams because the solid form of
boric acid was used and the solution desired was
expressed in metric units.

⊕ PREPARING A SOLUTION FROM A STOCK SOLUTION

EXAMPLE: Prepare 250 mL of a 5.0% solution from a 50% solution.

Formula: $\dfrac{D}{H} \times Q = x$

$\dfrac{5\%}{\cancel{50.0\%}_1} \times \cancel{250}^{5} \text{ mL} = 25 \text{ mL of solute needed}$

> *Answer* = The solution has a ratio strength of 1 : 10. Measure 25 mL of solute and add 225 mL of water to prepare 250 mL.

END OF CHAPTER REVIEW

Complete the following problems:

1. To prepare 400 mL of a 2% sodium bicarbonate solution from pure drug, you would need _____ grams of solute.

2. To make 1.5 L of a 5.0% solution from a 25% solution, you would need _____ mL of solute. Add _____ mL of water to make 1.5 L.

3. There is 500 mL of 40% magnesium sulfate solution available for a soak. To make a 30% solution, you would need _____ mL of solute. Add _____ mL of water to make 500 mL.

Solve the following drug administration problems and reduce each answer to its lowest terms.

1. Give 1.5 grams. The drug is available in 250-mg tablets. Give _____ tablet(s).

2. Give 2 teaspoons. The drug is available as 250 mg/5 mL. Give _____ mg.

3. Give 600 mg. The drug is available in 200-mg tablets. Give _____ tablet(s).

4. Give 0.3 grams. The drug is available as 150 mg/2.5 mL. Give _____ mL.

5. Give 75 mg. The drug is available as 25 mg/teaspoon. Give _____ mL.

6. Give 125 mg. The drug is available in 0.25-gram tablets. Give _____ tablet(s).

7. Give gr 1/100. Drug is available in 60-mg tablets. Give _____ tablet(s).

8. Give a liquid medication to a 6-month-old. The drug is available as 100 mg/5 mL for the normal adult daily dose. Give _____ mL/day.

9. Give 50 mg. The drug is available as 100 mg/2 mL. Give _____ mL.

10. Give 0.75 mg. The drug is available as 500 mcg/2mL. Give _____ mL.

11. Give gr iii. The drug is available as 60 mg/mL. Give _____ mL.

12. Give gr 1/8. The drug is available as 15 mg/mL. Give _____ mL.

13. Give 0.3 mg. The drug is available as 200 mcg/mL. Give _____ mL.

14. Give gr 1/6. The drug is available as 8 mg/mL. Give _____ mL.

15. Give 0.25 grams. The drug is available as 300 mg/2 mL. Give _____ mL.

Answer the next three questions by referring to the corresponding drug labels.

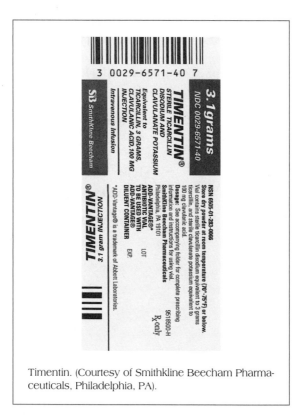

Timentin. (Courtesy of Smithkline Beecham Pharmaceuticals, Philadelphia, PA).

16. The physician prescribed Timentin 3.1 grams, IV, every 6 hours for a patient with a severe infection. The patient would receive _____ g of Timentin in 24 hours.

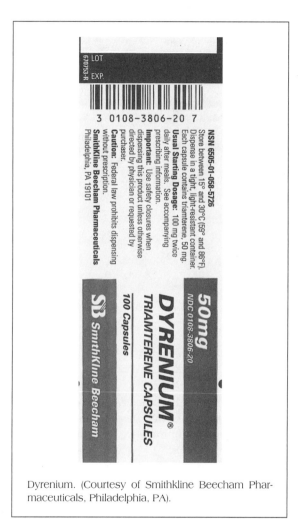

Dyrenium. (Courtesy of Smithkline Beecham Pharmaceuticals, Philadelphia, PA).

17. The physician prescribed Dyrenium 50 milligrams twice a day. The patient would receive _____ mg in 24 hours.

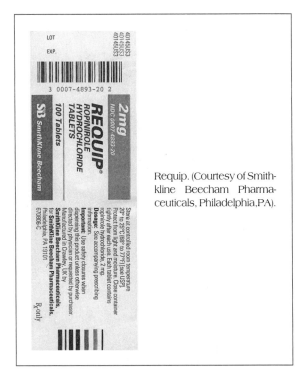

Requip. (Courtesy of Smith-Kline Beecham Pharmaceuticals, Philadelphia, PA).

18. A patient with Parkinson's disease is to receive Requip, 2 mg, three times a day. The nurse would administer _____ tablet(s) each dose for a total of _____ mg in 24 hours.

Solve the following drug administration problems and reduce the answers.

19. Give 500 mg of a medication that is available as a powder in a 2-gram vial. Reconstitute it by adding 11.5 mL of sterile water for injection. Each 1.5 mL of solution contains 250 mg of the medication. Give _____ mL.

20. Give 1 gram of a medication that is available as a powder in a 2-gram vial. Reconstitute it by adding 5 mL to achieve a concentration of 330 mg/mL. Give _____ mL.

21. Give 125 mg of a drug dissolved in 100 mL of a solution over 30 minutes. You would give _____ mL/h.

22. Give 1000 mL of a solution over 8 hours, using a drop factor of 10 gtt/mL. Give _____ gtt/min.

23. Give 500 mL of a solution over 10 hours, using a drop factor of 60 gtt/mL. Give _____ gtt/min.

24. Give 1000 mL of a solution over 6 hours, using a drop factor of 15 gtt/min. Give _____ gtt/min.

25. Give 800 mL of a solution at 12 gtt/min, using a drop factor of 10 gtt/min. Give over _____ hours and _____ min.

26. Give 250 mg of a solution in 500 mL at 10
    mL/h. Give _____ mg/h or _____ mcg/min.

27. Give 15 units of U-100 regular insulin by
    subcutaneous injection. Use U-100 regular
    insulin and a U-100 syringe. Draw up
    insulin in the syringe to the _____ unit
    marking.

28. Give 35 units of NPH and 10 units of regular
    insulin, using U-100 insulins and syringes.
    Draw up _____ units of _____ first,
    followed by _____ units of _____ .

29. Give 2,500 units of heparin subcutaneously.
    Vial concentration is 5,000 units/mL. Give
    _____ mL.

30. Give 1000 mL of D5W with 15,000 units of
    heparin to infuse at 30 mL/h. Give _____
    units/hour.

31. Give 800 units/h of heparin IV. Consider that
    500 mL of D5W is available, with 20,000
    units of heparin added. The drop factor is 60
    gtt/min. Give _____ gtt/min.

32. Give 1,000 mL of D5W with 40,000 units of
    heparin to infuse at 25 mL/h. Give _____
    units/h, which *is* or *is not* a safe dose. _____

33. Give 0.5 mL of IPV vaccine subcutaneously.
    A 5-mL multiple-dose vial is available. Give
    _____ mL. The vial contains a total of
    _____ doses.

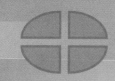

ANSWERS

CHAPTER 1

BASIC MATH PRETEST: Pages 3–8

1. viii   2. xiii   3. iiss̄
4. xxxvii   5. Li

6. 11 1/2   7. 16   8. 65
9. 9   10. 19

11. 5/8   12. 1/2   13. 1/2
14. 4/15

15. 1/3   16. 1/150   17. 1/100
18. 3/4

19. 3/8   20. 8 2/5   21. 3/4
22. 6 1/8   23. 1/60   24. 3 3/7
25. 1/48   26. 2/5

27. 14/5   28. 27/4   29. 94/9
30. 57/7

31. 3   32. 4 1/18   33. 3 2/11
34. 1 3/13

35. 0.33   36. 0.40   37. 0.37
38. 0.75

39. 1.81   40. 4.00   41. 5.87
42. 2.13

43. 48.78   44. 0.250   45. 72
46. 3.4

47. 1/4   48. 4/5   49. 1/3
50. 9/20   51. 3/4   52. 3/5
53. 3   54. 16   55. 2.6
56. 10   57. 0.75   58. 12
59. 24   60. 0.16   61. 0.9
62. 0.2

63. 20%	64. 36%	65. 7%
66. 12.5%	67. 10.3%	68. 183%
69. 25%	70. 60%	71. 1%
72. 198%	73. 120%	74. 14.2%
75. 0.25	76. 0.40	77. 0.80
78. 0.15	79. 0.048	80. 0.0036
81. 0.0175	82. 0.0830	

83. 18	84. 9	85. 1.08
86. 40	87. 25	88. 25%
89. 20%	90. 25%	91. 50
92. 120		

	Percent	Ratio	Common Fraction	Decimal
93.	25%	25 : 100	1/4	0.25
94.	3.3%	1 : 30	1/30	0.033
95.	5%	5 : 100	1/20	0.05
96.	0.67%	1 : 150	1/150	0.0067
97.	0.45%	45 : 100	9/20	0.0045
98.	1%	1 : 100	1/100	0.01
99.	0.83%	1 : 120	1/120	0.0083
100.	50%	50 : 100	1/2	0.50

CHAPTER 2

Practice Problems: Page 12

1. s̄s̄	2. iii	3. vii
4. x	5. xv	6. xxx
7. 6	8. 2	9. 5
10. 9	11. 20	12. 25

End of Chapter Review: Pages 12–13

1. xxvii	2. xxxii	3. xvi
4. iv	5. viii	6. x
7. xii	8. xxi	9. xviii

10. xxiv	11. 18	12. 16
13. 1/2	14. 9	15. 7 1/2
16. 19	17. 24	18. 14
19. 26	20. 6	

CHAPTER 3

Practice Problems: Page 15

1. $\dfrac{4 - N}{5 - D}$ 2. $\dfrac{1 - N}{2 - D}$ 3. $\dfrac{3 - N}{8 - D}$

4. $\dfrac{4 - N}{9 - D}$ 5. $\dfrac{7 - N}{8 - D}$ 6. $\dfrac{1 - N}{6 - D}$

Practice Problems: Pages 15–16

1. 7, 1/8	2. 9, 1/10	3. 4, 1/5
4. 3, 1/4	5. 2, 1/7	

Practice Problems: Page 18

1/300, 1/150, 1/100, 1/75, 1/25, 1/12, 1/9, 1/7, 1/3

Practice Problems: Pages 20–21

1. 69/12	2. 55/8	3. 43/5
4. 136/9	5. 98/3	6. 87/4
7. 37/2	8. 57/9	9. 27/5
10. 67/6		

Practice Problems: Page 22

1. 7 1/2	2. 6 5/6	3. 7 5/9
4. 6 6/11	5. 7 1/2	6. 2 2/3
7. 4 3/10	8. 7 3/4	9. 9 5/9
10. 18 2/3		

Practice Problems: Pages 24–25

1. 12/20   2. 20/40   3. 2/4
4. 5/8   5. 3/5   6. 6/10
7. 1/6   8. 1/6   9. 1/4
10. 1/18

Practice Problems: Page 27

1. 1/6   2. 1/6   3. 1/9

Practice Problems: Page 36

1. 2 5/11   2. 13/16   3. 3 19/24
4. 1 2/45   5. 1 3/10   6. 3/7
7. 4/9   8. 13/30   9. 19/36
10. 5 16/21

Practice Problems: Pages 40–41

1. 14/45   2. 5/21   3. 3/20
4. 1 7/20   5. 21/32   6. 6 3/4
7. 1 2/13   8. 1 5/9   9. 36
10. 29/50

End of Chapter Review: Pages 41–42

1. 14/35, 15/35   2. 28/20, 4/20
3. 1/6   4. 1/8   5. 6 1/2
6. 13 1/8   7. 50/11   8. 209/23
9. 5/16   10. 1/8   11. 1/9
12. 8/9   13. 1 1/3   14. 31/36
15. 7 5/24   16. 1/6   17. 5/9
18. 7/12   19. 4 9/40   20. 2 1/8
21. 3/20   22. 3/11   23. 14
24. 8   25. 6/11   26. 1 5/7
27. 24   28. 10 4/15   29. 5/56
30. 80

CHAPTER 4

Practice Problems: Pages 45–46

1. ten and one thousandths
2. three and seven ten-thousandths
3. eighty-three thousandths
4. one hundred fifty-three thousandths
5. thirty-six and sixty-seven ten-thousandths
6. one hundred twenty-five ten-thousandths
7. one hundred twenty-five and twenty-five thousandths
8. twenty and seventy-five thousandths
9. 5.037   10. 64.07   11. 0.020
12. 0.4   13. 8.064   14. 33.7
15. 0.015   16. 0.1

Practice Problems: Pages 54–55

1. 38.2   2. 18.409   3. 84.641
4. 243.58   5. 51.06   6. 12.33
7. 22.506   8. 6.8085   9. 101.4
10. 1065   11. 708.8   12. 30.538
13. 0.0984 14. 0.0008

Practice Problems: Pages 58–59

1. 0.20   2. 0.125   3. 0.25
4. 0.066   5. 0.066   6. 7/1000
7. 93/100   8. 103/250 9. 5 3/100
10. 12 1/5

End of Chapter Review: Pages 59–60

1. five and four hundredths
2. ten and sixty-five hundredths
3. eight thousandths

4. 6.08   5. 124.3   6. 16.001
7. 24.45   8. 59.262   9. 2.776
10. 5.210

11. 224.515   12. 0.1278   13. 1.56
14. 5.35   15. 0.60   16. 0.40
17. 0.142   18. 0.22   19. 0.75
20. 0.80   21. 9/20   22. 6 4/5
23. 3/4   24. 1 7/20   25. 3/50
26. 8 1/2

CHAPTER 5

Practice Problems: Page 65

1. 3/20   2. 3/10   3. 1/2
4. 3/4   5. 1/4   6. 3/5
7. 33⅓%   8. 66.6%   9. 20%
10. 75%   11. 40%   12. 25%

Practice Problems: Page 68

1. 0.15   2. 0.25   3. 0.59
4. 0.80   5. 25%   6. 45%
7. 60%   8. 85%

Practice Problems: Pages 78–79

1. $\dfrac{50 \text{ milligrams}}{5 \text{ milliliters}}$; 50 mg : 5 mL; 50 mg/5mL

2. $\dfrac{325 \text{ milligrams}}{1 \text{ tablet}}$; 325 mg : 1 tab; 325 mg/1 tab

3. $\dfrac{2 \text{ ampules}}{1 \text{ liter}}$; 2 amps : 1 L; 2 amps/1 L

4. $\dfrac{1 \text{ tablet}}{5 \text{ grains}}$: $\dfrac{3 \text{ tablets}}{15 \text{ grains}}$
   1 tab : 5 gr :: 3 tabs : 15 gr

5. $\dfrac{0.2 \text{ milligrams}}{1 \text{ tablet}} :: \dfrac{0.4 \text{ milligrams}}{2 \text{ tablets}}$

   0.2 mg : 1 tab :: 0.4 mg : 2 tabs

6. $\dfrac{10 \text{ milligrams}}{5 \text{ milliliters}} :: \dfrac{30 \text{ milligrams}}{15 \text{ milliliters}}$

   10 mg : 5mL :: 30 mg : 15 mL

7. $x = 9$

8. $x = 18$

9. $x = 4$

10. $\dfrac{50 \text{ mg}}{1 \text{ mL}} = \dfrac{40}{x \text{ mL}}$

    $50\,x = 40 \qquad x = 0.8 \text{ mL}$

11. $\dfrac{25 \text{ mg}}{1 \text{ mL}} = \dfrac{x \text{ mg}}{1.5 \text{ mL}}$

    $x = 25 \times 1.5 \qquad x = 37.5 \text{ mg}$

12. $\dfrac{0.125 \text{ mg}}{1 \text{ tablet}} = \dfrac{x}{2 \text{ tablets}}$

    $x = 0.125 \times 2 \qquad x = 0.25 \text{ mg}$

End of Chapter Review: Pages 79–83

	Percent	Fraction	Decimal
1.	16.6%	1/6	0.166
2.	25%	1/4	0.25
3.	6.4%	8/125	0.064
4.	21%	21/100	0.21
5.	40%	2/5	0.40
6.	162%	1 31/50	1.62
7.	27%	27/100	0.27
8.	5 1/4%	13/250	0.052
9.	450%	9/2	4.50
10.	8 1/3%	1/12	0.083
11.	1%	1/100	0.01

12.	85.7%	6/7	0.857
13.	450%	18/4	4.5
14.	150%	1 1/2	1.5
15.	72%	18/25	0.72

16. $\dfrac{10 \text{ mg}}{1 \text{ tab}}$; 10 mg : 1 tab

17. $\dfrac{10 \text{ units}}{1 \text{ mL}}$; 10 units : 1 mL

18. $\dfrac{200 \text{ mg}}{1 \text{ kilogram}}$; 200 mg : kg

19. $\dfrac{100 \text{ mg}}{1 \text{ tab}} :: \dfrac{300 \text{ mg}}{x \text{ tab}}$

  100 mg : 1 tab :: 300 mg : x tab

20. $\dfrac{250 \text{ mg}}{1 \text{ tab}} :: \dfrac{500 \text{ mg}}{x \text{ tab}}$

  250 mg : 1 tab :: 500 mg : x tab

21. $\dfrac{0.075 \text{ mg}}{1 \text{ tab}} :: \dfrac{0.15 \text{ mg}}{x \text{ tab}}$

  0.075 mg : 1 tab :: 0.15 mg : x tab

22. $\dfrac{4}{5}$ or 0.8

23. 6

24. 4.5

25. $x = 6$

26. 20 mg : 1 mL :: 10 mg : x mL

  20 mg $\times$ x mL = 10 mg $\times$ 1 mL

  $20x = 10$

  $\dfrac{20^1 x}{20_1} = \dfrac{10^1}{20_2} = \dfrac{1}{2} \; x = \dfrac{1}{2}$ mL

  $$Answer = \dfrac{1}{2} \text{ mL}$$

Verify the answer:

$$
\overbrace{20 \text{ mg} : 1 \text{ mL} :: 10 \text{ mg} : \underbrace{\tfrac{1}{2} (0.5) \text{ mL}}}^{\text{EXTREMES}}_{\text{MEANS}}
$$

$20 \text{ mg} \times 0.5 \text{ mL} = 10 \text{ mg} \times 1 \text{ mL}$

$20 \times 0.5 = 10$ Sum products

$10 \times 1 = 10$ are equal

27. $\dfrac{50 \text{ mg}}{5 \text{ mL}} = \dfrac{25 \text{ mg}}{x \text{ mL}}$

Cross-multiply:

$50 \text{ mg} \times x \text{ mL} = 25 \text{ mg} \times 5 \text{ mL}$

$50x = 125$

$$
\dfrac{\cancel{50}^{1} \, x}{\cancel{50}_{1}} = \dfrac{\cancel{125}^{5}}{\cancel{50}_{2}}
$$

$x = \dfrac{5}{2} = 2\dfrac{1}{2} \text{ mL}$

Answer = 2.5 mL

Verify the answer:

$\dfrac{50 \text{ mg}}{5 \text{ mL}} = \dfrac{25}{2.5 \text{ mL}}$

$50 \times 2.5 = 125$ Sum products

$25 \times 5 = 125$ are equal

28. $3.0 \text{ mg} : 1.0 \text{ mL} :: 1.5 \text{ mg} : x \text{ mL}$

$3.0 \text{ mg} \times x \text{ mL} = 1.5 \text{ mg} \times 1.0 \text{ mL}$

$3x = 1.5$

$$\frac{\overset{1}{\cancel{3}}x}{\cancel{3}_1} = \frac{\overset{1}{\cancel{1.5}}}{\cancel{3}_2} = \frac{1}{2}$$

$$x = \frac{1}{2} \text{ mL}$$

$$Answer = \frac{1}{2} \text{ mL}$$

Verify the answer:

┌────EXTREMES────┐

3.0 mg : 1.0 mL :: 1.5 mg : 0.5 mL

└─ MEANS ─┘

3.0 mg × 0.5 mL = 1.5 mg × 1.0 mL

3.0 × 0.5 = 1.5 ⎫ Sum products
1.5 × 1.0 = 1.5 ⎭ are equal

29. 20 mg : 2 mL :: 35 mg : x mL

20 mg × x mL = 35 mg × 2 mL

20x = 70

$$\frac{\overset{1}{\cancel{20}}x}{\cancel{20}^1} = \frac{70}{20} = \frac{7}{2} \; x = 3 \; 1/2 \text{ mL}$$

$$Answer = 3 \; 1/2 \text{ mL}$$

Verify the answer:

20 mg : 2 mL :: 35 mg : 3 1/2 mL

20 mg × 3.5 mL = 35 mg × 2 mL

20 × 3.5 = 70 ⎫ Sum products
35 × 2 = 70 ⎭ are equal

30. 7.5 mL
31. 7.5 mL
32. 0.5 mL
33. 1.5 mL
34. 1.6 mL

END OF UNIT I REVIEW: PAGES 84–85

1. 1
2. 1/15
3. 7/10
4. 5/12
5. 2 2/5
6. 1/16
7. 3 1/3
8. 1/150
9. 2
10. 4/5
11. 1/4
12. 3 1/3
13. 1/3
14. 1/6
15. 1/100
16. 5/30
17. 3.1
18. 4.26
19. 0.4
20. 5.68
21. 2.5
22. 15
23. 16.66
24. 1.88
25. 0.8
26. 0.25
27. 0.33
28. 1/2
29. 7/100
30. 1 1/2
31. 1/4
32. 1/300
33. 3/500
34. 40%
35. 450%
36. 2%
37. 12
38. 1 1/5
39. 1 1/4
40. 1 3/5
41. 1/2
42. 15

CHAPTER 6

Practice Problems: Page 93

1. 0.0360 m
2. 41.6 dm
3. 0.08 cm
4. 0.002 m

Practice Problems: Page 95

1. 0.003006 L   2. 61.7 mL
3. 900 mL   4. 64 mg
5. 1.0 g   6. 0.008 dg

End of Chapter Review: Page 96

1. 0.00743 m   2. 0.006 dm
3. 10,000 m   4. 6217 mm
5. 0.0164 dL   6. 0.047 L
7. 1000 cL   8. 569 mL
9. 0.0356 g   10. 30 cg
11. 50 mg   12. 930 mg
13. 0.1 mg   14. 2000 mcg
15. 0.001 mg   16. 7000 g
17. 4000 mcg   18. 13,000 g
19. 2500 mL   20. 600 mcg
21. 80 mg   22. 10 mcg

CHAPTER 7

End of Chapter Review: Page 101

1. gr iii   2. ʒ v   3. fʒ vii
4. mx   5. mxxss̄
6. pt v   7. 2   8. 960 m
9. 32   10. 1/2   11. 1
12. 2   13. 1/4 pt   14. ʒ 1/4
15. ʒ ii   16. ʒ iv

CHAPTER 8

End of Chapter Review: Page 108

1. 2 cups	2. 24 oz	3. 3 oz
4. 120 gtt	5. 9 tsp	6. 12 oz
7. 1/2 pt	8. 1 pt	9. 4 T
10. 2 oz	11. 6 oz	12. 1.5 qt
13. 1 oz	14. 32 oz	15. 30 gtt

CHAPTER 9

Practice Problems: Pages 113–114

1. 48–60 mL	2. 45–48 m
3. 8–10 mL	4. 0.3 mg
5. 24–30 g	6. 1 ounce
7. gr 1/10	8. 1 quart
9. 1 kg	

End of Chapter Review: Pages 114–116

1. 25 kg	2. 60 g
3. 960 mL	4. 4 inches
5. 1 tsp	6. 300–325 mg
7. 3 gtt	8. gr 1/150
9. ℥ viii	10. 300 mcg or 0.3 mg
11. 1.8 g	12. 2 oz
13. 6 tablets	14. 1 tsp; f℥ 1
15. 15 mL or 3 teaspoons	16. 0.4 gram
17. 125 mg; 1 g	18. 450 mL

END OF UNIT II REVIEW: Page 117

1. 80 mg	2. 3,200 mL
3. 1.5 mg	4. 125 mcg

5. 20,000 g	6. 0.005 g
7. 4 drams	8. ℥s̈s̈
9. 1/4	10. 16 ounces
11. 1 1/2 quarts	12. ℥ İ
13. 3 teaspoons	14. 1 ounce
15. 6 ounces	16. 1 ounce
17. 30 mg	18. 1 ounce
19. 30 mL	20. 60–65 mg
21. 15 mL	22. 44 pounds
23. 0.4 mg	24. gr 1/200

CHAPTER 10

Practice Problems: Page 125

1. Ropinirole hydrochloride
2. NDC 0007-4893-20
3. 2 mg
4. 100 tablets
5. Tablets

End of Chapter Review: Pages 129–133

1. 1 tablet; 1200 mg
2. 500 mg; 0.5 grams
3. 2.5 mL; 300 mg; 7.5 mL
4. 1 tablet; 40 mg
5. 2 vials
6. 2 mL

CHAPTER 11

Practice Problems: Pages 138–140

1. 4 tablets	2. 15 mL
3. 1/2 tablet	4. 10 mL

5. 3 tablets
6. 2 tablets
7. 5 mL
8. 1/2 tablet
9. 3/5 tablet
10. 4 tablets
11. 3 tablets
12. 12 mL
13. 15 mL
14. 10 mL
15. 2 tablets
16. 12.5 mL
17. 8 tablets
18. 8–10 mL
19. 3 tablets
20. 4 tablets
21. 2 tablets

Practice Problems: Pages 143–144

1. 15 mL; 30 mg
2. 1/2 tsp; 7.5 mL
3. gr 1/60
4. 18.8 mL
5. 2 tablets
6. 2 tablets
7. 1 tablet
8. 2 tsp
9. 1 tablet
10. 10 mL; 2 tsp
11. 15 mL; 1/2 oz
12. 2 capsules

End of Chapter Review: Pages 154–157

1. 3 tablets
2. 3 tablets
3. 30 mL
4. 4 tablets
5. 1 tablet
6. 2 tablets
7. 1 ounce
8. 1 tablet
9. 7.5 mL
10. 1 tablet
11. 1 tablet; 4 tablets
12. 4 tablets
13. 4 tablets
14. 1 tsp; 3 i
15. 10 mL; 2 tsp
16. 50 mg
17. 4 tablets
18. 2 tablets
19. 1 tablet
20. 250 mg
21. 30 mg in 0.6 mL
22. 10 mg in 4 mL
23. 0.8 mg in 2 mL
24. 20 mg
25. Surface area = 1.0 m² Dosage = 29 mg
   divided into 4 equal doses of 7.25 mg every
   6 hours

CHAPTER 12

Practice Problems: Page 166

1. 2 mL   2. 4 mL   3. 3 mL
4. 3 mL   5. 0.8 mL

End of Chapter Review: Pages 167–171

1. 2.5 mL	2. 0.4 mL	3. 0.75 mL
4. 0.7 mL	5. 3 mL	6. 0.6 mL
7. 0.75 mL	8. 0.75 mL	9. 1.25 mL
10. 1 mL	11. 0.8 mL	12. 1.8 mL
13. 0.75 mL	14. 0.5 mL	15. 0.6 mL
16. 2 mL	17. 0.5 mL	18. 1.5 mL
19. 1.5 mL	20. 0.8 mL	21. 1.8 mL
22. 3 mL	23. 2 mL	24. 0.1 mL
25. 0.5 mL	26. 0.8 mL	27. 0.5 mL

CHAPTER 13

Practice Problems: Pages 184–186

1. 83 mL/h	2. 125 mL/h
3. 27 gtt/min	4. 42 gtt/min
5. 21 gtt/min	6. 17 gtt/min
7. 17 gtt/min	8. 19 gtt/min
9. 20 gtt/min	10. 38 gtt/min
11. 19 gtt/min	12. 17 gtt/min
13. 25 gtt/min	14. 67 gtt/min

End of Chapter Review, Pages 192–196

1. 63 mL/h	2. 100 mL/h
3. 250 mL/h	4. 83 mL/h
5. 50 mL/h	6. 63 mL/h
7. 21 gtt/min	8. 42 gtt/min
9. 167 mL/h;	10. 10 gtt/min
28 gtt/min	
11. 19 gtt/min	
12. 8 gtt/min	13. 20 h
14. 12 1/2 h	15. 12 1/2 h
16. 13 gtt/min	17. 42 gtt/min
18. 38 gtt/min	19. 100 gtt/min
20. 30 gtt/min	21. 70 gtt/min; 70 mL
22. 200 mcg/mL;	23. 0.7 mL
67–68 mL/h	
24. 2 mL; 30 mL/h	25. 125 mL
26. 3.0 mL	27. 18 mL/h; 18 mg/h
28. 10 gtt/min	29. 0.5 mL
30. 15 gtt/min	31. 40 gtt/min; 40 mL
32. 100 mL/h;	
34 gtt/min	

CHAPTER 14

Practice Problems: Pages 204–205

1. 60 U of U-100

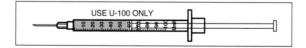

2. 82 U of U-100

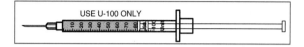

3. 45 U of U-100

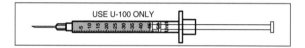

4. 35 U of U-100

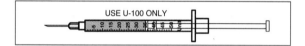

5. 26 U of U-100

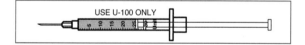

6. 56 U of U-100

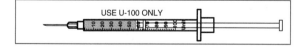

7. 60 U   8. 40 U
9. 20 U   10. 70 U
11. 21; U-30/0.5 mL   12. 45; U-50/0.5 mL
13. 64; U-100/1 mL   14. 38; U-50/0.5 mL
15. 56; U-100/1 mL

Practice Problems: Pages 215–216

1. 400 U/h; safe
2. 20 mL/h
3. 20 mL/h; 20 gtt/min

End of Chapter Review: Pages 217–220

1. U-50; 30 U   2. 39 U; U-50
3. 15 U   4. 50 U
5. 34 U; NPH   6. 3; 2 U
7. 0.6 mL; 20,000 U;   8. 0.8 mL; 24,000 U;
   is within   is within
9. 0.6 mL; 10,000 U;   10. 0.25 mL
   is within
11. 600 U/h   12. 1.5 mL/min = 90
13. 50 mL/h;   mL/h; 1,350 U/h =
    17 gtt/min   32,400 U/24 h
14. 1.2 mL   15. 0.5 mL
16. 2.5 mL   17. 4 mL
18. 21 mL/hr; 625 U/h   19. 6 gtt/min
20. 32 units; U-50

CHAPTER 15

End of Chapter Review: Pages 222–223

1. 0.5 mL   2. 0.5 mL   3. 8.8 mL
4. 2 mL   5. 12.5 mL   6. 3 mL
7. 13.5 mL   8. 0.5 mL   9. 3.6 mL

10. 0.5 mL; 20 doses   11. 0.5 mL

CHAPTER 16

End of Chapter Review: Page 227

1. 8 grams
2. 300 mL; 1200 mL
3. 375 mL; 125 mL

END OF UNIT III REVIEW: PAGES 228–234

1. 6 tablets
2. 500 mg
3. 3 tablets
4. 5 mL
5. 15 mL
6. 1/2 tablet
7. 1 tablet
8. 2 mL
9. 1 mL
10. 3 mL
11. 30 mL
12. 0.5 mL
13. 1.5 mL
14. 1.25 mL
15. 1.66 mL
16. 12.4 grams
17. 100 mg
18. 1 tablet; 6 mg
19. 3 mL
20. 3 mL
21. 200 mL
22. 21 gtt/min
23. 50 gtt/min (approximate)
24. 41.6 gtt/min (approximate)
25. 11 hours; 6 min
26. 5 mg/h; 83 mcg/min
27. 15
28. 10 units of regular; 35 units of NPH
29. 0.5 mL
30. 450 units/h
31. 20 gtt/min
32. 1,000 units/h; a safe dose
33. 0.5 mL/10 doses

APPENDIX A

Rounding Off Decimals

> ► RULE: To round off decimals, follow these steps:

- Determine the place that the decimal is to be "rounded off" to (tenths, hundredths). For example, let's round off 36.315 to the nearest hundredth.
- Bracket the number [ ] in the hundredths place (2 places to the right of the decimal). For 36.315, you would bracket the 1. Then 36.315 would look like this 36.3[1]5.
- Look at the number to the right of the bracket. For 36.3[1]5, that number would be 5.
- If the number to the right of the bracket is less than 5 (< 5), then drop the number. If it is 5 or greater than 5 (> 5), then increase the bracketed number by 1.

For 36.3[1]5, increase the bracketed number [1] by 1. The rounded off number becomes 36.32.

EXAMPLE: 5.671

5.6[7]1

Look at the number to the right of [7].

The number is < 5.

Leave [7] as is; drop 1.

[7] stays as [7].

5.671 rounds off to 5.67.

Answer = 5.67

Intradermal Injections

The *intradermal route* is preferred for:

- Small quantities of medication (0.1 mL–0.2 mL)
- Nonirritating solutions that are slowly absorbed
- Allergy testing
- PPD administration (screening for tuberculosis)

The Intradermal Route

Use
A tuberculin syringe

Inject
Into dermis or upper layer of tissue under the outer layer of skin or epidermis. Make sure the bevel of the needle is up.

Angle
15 degrees   15° ↑

Administering an Intradermal Injection

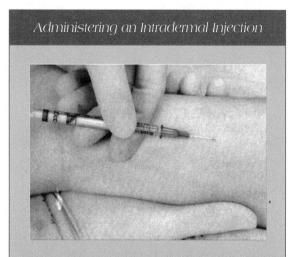

Inserting the needle almost level with the skin. (From Taylor, C., Lillis, C., and LeMone, P. [2001]: *Fundamentals of nursing: The art and science of nursing care* [4th ed.]. Philadelphia: Lippincott Williams & Wilkins, p. 598.)

Gauge		Needle Length		Solution	
Range	Average	Range	Average	Range	Average
27–25	26	$\frac{3}{8} - \frac{5}{8}$	$\frac{1}{2}$	0.1 mL–0.5 mL	0.1 mL

Subcutaneous Injections

The Subcutaneous Route

Use
- An insulin syringe
- A prefilled disposable syringe with appropriate needle length

Inject
Under the skin into the fibrous tissue above the muscle

*Angle**
45–90 degrees

45°   90°

*A 45-degree angle of insertion is used with a 5/8" needle for subcutaneous medications *except insulin and heparin,* for example, codeine sulfate and oxymorphone hydrochloride. A 90-degree angle of insertion is used with a 3/8"–1/2" needle for *insulin and heparin.*

Administering a Subcutaneous Injection

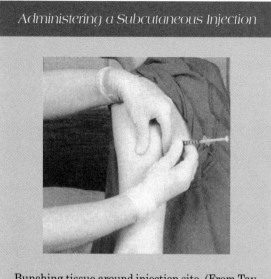

Bunching tissue around injection site. (From Taylor, C., Lillis, C., and LeMone, P. [2001]: *Fundamentals of nursing: The art and science of nursing care,* [4th ed.]. Philadelphia: Lippincott Williams & Wilkins, p. 601.)

Gauge		Needle Length		Solution	
Range	Average	Range	Average	Range	Average
27–25	26	$\frac{3}{8} - \frac{5}{8}$	$\frac{3}{8} - \frac{1}{2}$ $\bar{c}$ 90° $\frac{5}{8}$ $\bar{c}$ 45°	0.2 mL– 2.0 mL	<0.1 mL

Intramuscular Injections

The *intramuscular route* is preferred for medications that:

- Are irritating to subcutaneous tissue
- Require a rapid rate of absorption
- Can be administered in volumes up to 5.0 mL

The Intramuscular Route

Use
A 3.0 mL–5.0 mL syringe

Inject
Into the body of a striated muscle. Inject past the dermis and subcutaneous tissue. Always aspirate before injecting.

Angle
Always 90 degrees

↓ 90°

Administering an Intramuscular Injection

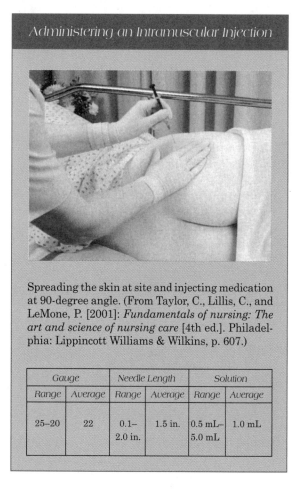

Spreading the skin at site and injecting medication at 90-degree angle. (From Taylor, C., Lillis, C., and LeMone, P. [2001]: *Fundamentals of nursing: The art and science of nursing care* [4th ed.]. Philadelphia: Lippincott Williams & Wilkins, p. 607.)

Gauge		Needle Length		Solution	
Range	Average	Range	Average	Range	Average
25–20	22	0.1–2.0 in.	1.5 in.	0.5 mL–5.0 mL	1.0 mL

Z-Track Injections

The *Z-track* method is used for parenteral drug administration when tissue damage from the leakage of irritating medications is expected or when it is essential that all of the medication can be absorbed in the muscle and not in the subcutaneous tissue. The method is easy, popular, and recommended by some institutions as a safe way of administering all intramuscular injections. This method prevents "tracking" of the medication along the path of the needle during insertion and removal.

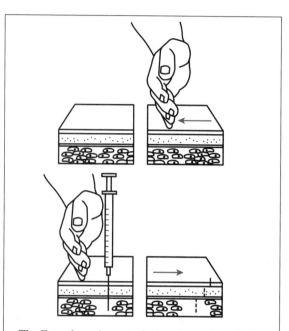

The Z-track or zigzag technique is used to administer medications that are irritating to subcutaneous tissue. The skin is pulled to one side. The needle is aspirated for blood by pulling back on the plunger, and the solution is injected. When the needle is withdrawn and the displaced tissue is allowed to return to its normal position, the solution is prevented from escaping from the muscle tissue. (From Taylor, C., Lillis, C., and LeMone, P. [2001]: *Fundamentals of nursing: The art and science of nursing care,* [4th ed.]. Philadelphia: Lippincott Williams & Wilkins, p. 608.)

The Z-Track Route

Use
A 3.0–5.0 mL syringe

Inject
Deep into the body of the gluteal muscle; the vastus lateralis can also be used.

Angle
Always 90 degrees

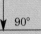

90°

Injection Technique
Displace or push tissue over muscle toward the center of the body by displacing the tissue with the last three fingers of the nondominant hand. Hold the tissues in this displaced position before, during, and for 5 to 15 seconds after the injection so the medication can begin to be absorbed. Use the IM injection technique as described on page 262.

Pediatric Intramuscular Injections

The Intramuscular Route

Use
A needle about 1 inch in length. For infants a 5/8"
needle may be used.

Inject
Into dense muscle mass in the deltoid and ven-
trogluteal muscles. Into the outer quadrant of the
gluteal and vastus lateralis muscles.

Angle
Preferably 45 degrees. May use 90 degrees if child's
age and body mass warrant it.

Injection Technique
Similar to the intramuscular technique for adults
as described on page 262.

Gauge		Needle Length		Solution	
Range	Average	Range	Average	Range	Average
22–20	22	0.5 in– 1.5 in	1.0 in	0.5 mL– 2.5 mL	0.5–1.0 < 3 yrs 0.5–1.5 4–6 yrs 0.5–2.0 7–14 yrs 1.0–2.5 > 15 yrs

APPENDIX G

Nursing Concerns for Pediatric Drug Administration

When administering medications to children, you need to be aware of the following:

- Explain honestly what will be done; explain at the level of the child's understanding.
- Use supplemental materials to promote understanding (stuffed animals, dolls).
- Suggest that the child help as much as possible; encourage the child to pretend and switch roles with the child.
- Reinforce positive behavior with praise and rewards if necessary.
- Make sure you have obtained an accurate height and weight measurement.
- Be sure that you have compared the normal dose range with the dosage you plan to give; know toxic and lethal doses.
- Do not force medication on a frightened child, especially one who is crying.
- Always use two people when giving injections to small children.
- Disguise or dilute medications if necessary.

A nurse also needs to understand that the child's immature body systems may respond differently to drugs, so there may be changes in an agent's absorption, distribution, biotransformation, and elimination. (See Appendix F for information about pediatric intramuscular injections.)

Nursing Concerns for Geriatric Drug Administration

As with pediatric medications, special considera-
tion is given when administering drugs to anyone
who is over 65 years. This is because physiological
changes caused by aging change the way the body
reacts to certain drugs. For example, a tranquilizer may increase restlessness and agitation in an
elderly person.

You should be aware of the following general
considerations before administering a drug to any
elderly individual.

- Small, frail elderly individuals will probably
  require less than the normal adult dosages.
  Drug absorption and distribution are
  affected by decreased gastrointestinal
  motility, decreased muscle mass, and
  diminished tissue perfusion.
- A drug should be given orally rather than
  parenterally, if possible, because decreased
  activity in the elderly decreases muscle
  tissue absorption.
- Often, it will be necessary to crush pills,
  empty capsules, or dissolve medications in
  liquid in order to assist the person to
  swallow without discomfort. Tell the patient
  not to crush enteric-coated or time-released
  drugs.

- Sedatives and narcotics must be given with extreme caution to elderly people, for they may easily become oversedated.
- Because the elderly are often on many different medications, you should check for drug interactions that may cause hazardous effects (eg, giving a sedative shortly after a tranquilizer).
- The cumulative side effects of the drugs being administered must be monitored. A drug's excretion may be altered if the patient has reduced renal blood flow and reduced kidney function.
- A schedule for rotation of injection sites should be followed carefully because the elderly have decreased muscle mass and increased vascular fragility.
- Any written directions for medication administration should be clear and in large print because of possible impaired vision.
- The problem of impaired hearing should be remembered when giving directions or asking questions. You may have to speak very loudly or repeat the same information several times. Writing the directions is recommended for some patients.
- Reinforce any important information by asking the patient to repeat it for you. This also helps you to ascertain whether the information was understood. Memory loss and confusion are common in the elderly because of cerebral arteriosclerosis.

Abbreviations and Symbols for Drug Preparation and Administration

ABBREVIATION/SYMBOL	INTERPRETATION
a or ā	before
@	at
aa or $\overline{aa}$	of each
a.c.	before meals
A.D.	right ear
ad lib.	as desired
A.L. or A.S.	left ear
alt. h.	alternate hour
aq.	water
A.S.A.P.	as soon as possible
A.U.	both ears
b.i.d.	twice a day
b.i.n.	twice a night
c	with
C	gallon
cap(s).	capsule(s)
cc	cubic centimeter
cm	centimeter
comp.	compound
conc.	concentrate
D/C	discontinue
dil.	dilute
disp.	dispense
dist.	distilled

ABBREVIATION/SYMBOL	INTERPRETATION
dr or ℥	dram
Dx	diagnose
elix.	elixir
et	and
ext.	extract; external
fl; fld	fluid
g	gram
gal	gallon
gm	gram
gr	grain
gtt	drops
h	hour
Ⓗ	hypodermic
h.s.	hour of sleep; at bedtime
ID	intradermal
IM	intramuscular
IV	intravenous
kg	kilogram
KVO	keep vein open
L	liter
lb	pound
M; m	meter
m; min	minim
mcg	microgram
mEq	milliequivalent
mg; mgm	milligram
mL	milliliter
mm	millimeter
noct.	at night
N.P.O.	nothing by mouth
NSS	normal saline solution
O.	pint
O.D.	right eye

ABBREVIATION/SYMBOL	INTERPRETATION
o.d.; q.d.	once every day
o.h.	every hour
o.m.	every morning
o.n.	every night
O.S.	left eye
OTC	over-the-counter
O.U.	both eyes
oz	ounce
$\bar{p}$	after
p.c.	after meals
per	by
p.o. or per os	by mouth
p.r.n.	as needed; when necessary
p.s.s.	physiologic saline solution
pt	pint
q	each; every
qh	every hour
q.i.d.	four times a day
q2h	every 2 hours
q3h	every 3 hours
q4h	every 4 hours
q6h	every 6 hours
q8h	every 8 hours
q12h	every 12 hours
q.o.d.	every other day
q.s.	quantity sufficient; as much as needed
qt	quart
R	rectally
℞	to take; by prescription
R/O	rule out

ABBREVIATION/SYMBOL	INTERPRETATION
s	without
SC, s.c.; s.q., sub q sub cut	subcutaneously
sig.	label; write
SL; subl.	sublingual
sol; soln	solution
s.o.s.	one dose as necessary
stat.	immediately
supp.	suppository
tab	tablet
tbs; T	tablespoon
t.i.d.	three times a day
tinct; tr	tincture
T.K.O.	to keep open
tsp; t	teaspoon
μg	microgram
ung.	ointment

Temperature Conversions: Fahrenheit and Celsius Scales

The Celsius scale is also known as the centigrade scale and is being used more often now that the metric system is becoming more popular. The Fahrenheit scale is used primarily for measuring body temperature.

> ► RULE: To change from Fahrenheit to Celsius, perform the following steps:

- Subtract 32 degrees from the Fahrenheit reading.
- Multiply by 5/9 or divide by 9/5 (1.8).

- $C = (F - 32) \times \dfrac{5}{9}$

EXAMPLE: Convert 100°F to Celsius.

$$
\begin{array}{c}
100 \\
\underline{-32} \\
68
\end{array}
\qquad
\frac{68}{1} \times \frac{5}{9} = \frac{340}{9}
$$

$$= 340 \div 9 = 37.7°C$$

Answer = 37.7° Celsius

> ➤ RULE: To change from Celsius to
>   Fahrenheit, perform the following steps:

- Multiply the Celsius reading by 9/5 or 1.8.
- Add 32

- $F = (9/5 \times C$ or $C \times 1.8) + 32$

EXAMPLE: Convert 40°C to Fahrenheit.

$$\cancel{40}^8 \times \frac{9}{\cancel{5}_1} = 72$$

or

$$40 \times 1.8 = 72$$

$$\begin{array}{r} 72 \\ +32 \\ \hline 104° \end{array}$$

Answer = 104° Fahrenheit

You may find the following temperature conversion scale useful for quick reference.

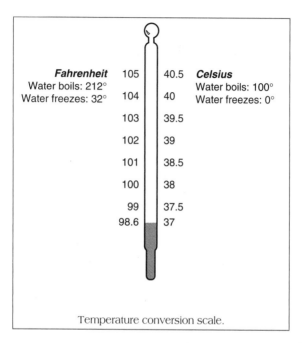

Temperature conversion scale.

Dosage Calculation Examples Using Dimensional Analysis

Nurses have used dimensional analysis (DA) to solve medication administration problems in nursing for about 30 years. The process is commonly referred to as the *factor method* because drug dosages are considered *factors* and calculations are solved using a *factor method*. The unit of measure is the drug form being calculated (eg, milliliter, tablet, capsule).

As a variation of ratio and proportion, DA has failed to achieve widespread use. It is presented here in abbreviated form as a reference for those who choose to use it. The following steps present a sample oral dosage calculation problem:

EXAMPLE: Give 500 mg of a drug twice daily. The drug is available as 0.25 grams per tablet.

> ➤ RULE: To prepare an oral dosage of a medication by using DA for calculations, follow these steps.

- ♦ List the unit of measure first, followed by an equal sign:

  Tab =

♦ Write the numerator of the first fraction, which must be the same unit of measurement as the unit to the left of the equal sign.

Tab = 1 tab

♦ Write the first denominator in the fraction. It is the factor that contains the unit of measure.

$$\text{Tab} = \frac{1\text{ tab}}{0.25\text{ grams}}$$

♦ The first fraction is called the "starting factor," and it is followed by the multiplication symbol (×) to set up a proportion format.

$$\text{Tab} = \frac{1\text{ tab}}{0.25\text{ grams}} \times$$

♦ The numerator of the second fraction must match the unit of measure in the first denominator. Therefore, the unit of measure "grams" must be in the numerator of the second fraction. Because 500 mg is the desired dose, 500 mg is changed to 0.5 grams.

$$\text{Tab} = \frac{1\text{ tab}}{0.25\text{ grams}} \times 0.5\text{ grams}$$

♦ Cancel the opposite and matching units of measure in the denominator and numerator. This verifies that they are similar and helps set up the fraction format to complete the mathematical calculations. Never cancel the unit of measure in the first numerator.

$$\text{Tab} = \frac{1\text{ tab}}{0.25\text{ \sout{grams}}} \times 0.5\text{ \sout{grams}}$$

♦ Complete the mathematical calculations.

$$\text{Tab} = \frac{1 \text{ tab}}{0.25} \times 0.5 = \frac{0.5}{0.25} = 2$$

$$Answer = 2 \text{ tablets}$$

EXAMPLE: Give 250 mg of a drug available as 0.5 grams per 2 mL. The following steps reiterate the rule on using DA.

♦ Write the unit of measure, followed by an equal sign:

$$\text{mL} =$$

♦ Add the numerator with a similar unit of measure and its associated factor for the denominator. Follow with a multiplication symbol ($\times$).

$$\text{mL} = \frac{2 \text{ mL}}{0.5 \text{ grams}} \times$$

♦ Write the second fraction, matching the unit of measure from the previous denominator. Because the drug is available in grams, it is best to convert milligrams to grams. Therefore, 250 mg equals 0.25 grams.

$$\text{mL} = \frac{2 \text{ mL}}{0.5 \text{ grams}} \times 0.25 \text{ grams}$$

♦ Complete the mathematical calculations.

$$\text{mL} = \frac{2 \text{ mL}}{0.5 \text{ \sout{grams}}} \times 0.25 \text{ \sout{grams}}$$

$$\frac{2 \text{ mL}}{0.5} \times 0.25 = \frac{0.25}{0.50} = \frac{1}{2} \times 2 \text{ mL} = 1 \text{ mL}$$

$$Answer = 1 \text{ mL}$$

Index

Page numbers followed by f indicate figures; n following a page number indicates footnoted material; t following a page number indicates tabular material.